*Next Medicine*

# Next Medicine

*The Science and Civics of Health*

Walter M. Bortz II, M.D.

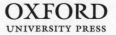

OXFORD
UNIVERSITY PRESS

2011

## OXFORD
UNIVERSITY PRESS

Oxford University Press, Inc., publishes works that further
Oxford University's objective of excellence
in research, scholarship, and education.

Oxford  New York
Auckland   Cape Town   Dar es Salaam   Hong Kong   Karachi
Kuala Lumpur   Madrid   Melbourne   Mexico City   Nairobi
New Delhi   Shanghai   Taipei   Toronto

With offices in
Argentina   Austria   Brazil   Chile   Czech Republic   France   Greece
Guatemala   Hungary   Italy   Japan   Poland   Portugal   Singapore
South Korea   Switzerland   Thailand   Turkey   Ukraine   Vietnam

Copyright © 2011 by Walter M. Bortz

Published by Oxford University Press, Inc.
198 Madison Avenue, New York, New York 10016
www.oup.com

Library of Congress Cataloging-in-Publication Data

Bortz, Walter M.
Next medicine : the science and civics of health/Walter M. Bortz II.
p. ; cm.
Includes bibliographical references and index.
ISBN 978-0-19-536968-7
1. Medical care—United States. 2. Medical technology—United States.
3. Health care reform—United States. 4. Medicine, Preventive—
United States. I. Title.
[DNLM: 1. Delivery of Health Care—trends—United States.
2. Biomedical Technology—trends—United States. 3. Health Care
Reform—United States. 4. Preventive Medicine—trends—
United States.  W 84 AA1 B739n 2011]
RA445.B67 2011
362.10973—dc22                    2010013587

3  5  7  9  8  6  4  2

Printed in the United States of America
on acid-free paper

*I dedicate this book to the renaissance of my profession.*

# Acknowledgments

This is the seventh book which I have written. The other six concerned the two primary devotions of my career, diabetes and aging. I enjoyed their creation, as they gave room to blend my clinical experience with the emerging science of both fields. They also provided gratification in that my efforts may have had effects beyond house calls, and office visits.

One such situation concerned a phone call which I received maybe six years ago. "Dr. Bortz. My name is Mary Morgan, and I got your name from a mutual friend who suggested that because of your long experience in the community you could help me affiliate with a new doctor, since I am recently moved here from out of state." Such calls are fairly common and represent a small nuisance, but I obligingly offered names of three family doctors, members of my Palo Alto Clinic, where I had practiced for 30 years.

A couple days later she called back. "Dr. Bortz, I contacted one of your suggested referrals and he said that he would accept me as a new patient if you would call him personally on my behalf." I hope that I did not reflect my irk, but replied "Okay, but I really don't know anything about you, who are you? Where do you come from? What are your medical problems?" She responded, "Of course, I'm from

New York City. I'm very healthy, and my husband was a prominent pediatrician back East."

"What was his name?"

"Spock."

"Benjamin Spock?"

"Yes."

"Why didn't you tell me that on your first call? Because any physician would be proud to serve Dr. Spock's widow. Your husband was a central feature of my life, almost a third parent in our raising of our four children through those nettlesome years."

She replied, "Dr. Bortz, that is very sweet of you, but I must tell you something. My husband read your books on aging and remarked how much you had helped him in his later years."

This totally unexpected encounter was immensely fulfilling, to consider that I, by reaching into the deep themes of life's terminus, might help the person who had done so much in getting our kids started out right.

My earlier books were gratifying in their circumscribed reach, but I felt a desire for a broader platform. I searched for the first principles from which all else derives, the *why* of my life. When I was young Granddaddy Bortz said to me dismissively, "Go make yourself necessary." As a youngster this remark meant "scat," but now at 80 years of age I find I must respond to Granddaddy by reaching out to the big lessons that life has taught.

My career as a physician has brought riches beyond counting, and I feel I'm just about the luckiest person in the world. But beyond this deep satisfaction which medicine has brought me, I now sorrow for its fall from grace. Mine is only one voice in recognizing this situation. Yet I feel that because of the breadth of my experience it may be helpful to propose constructive comment. In this I reference Albert St. Gyorgye's remark, "to see what all see, but say what none say." In my view most of the available commentary about medicine's distress are fragmentary at best, and represent baby steps when a leap is necessary. Someone commented that you cannot cross a chasm incrementally.

This book represents my major effort to survey the decades and continents of my life and learn from them lessons that might inform others beyond me. As I begin the accounting of those who have been my coworkers in this effort I identify immediately the impossibility of adequate response. I can fill 10 pages of tributes with no difficulty. Accordingly these acknowledgments must be generic in type. Of course I begin with family members who have been a constant sounding board for ideas good and bad. My patients are probably next in prioritizing my judgments. My colleagues, clinical, scientific, and administrative have been steadfast and immense in their generosities. And of course my institutional affiliations at the Palo Alto Medical Clinic and Stanford University School of Medicine have been central in my nurture. They daily expanded my horizons. In writing this book, international travel has extended and sustained my curiosity and modesty. Further, I intentionally returned to my underlines of thousands of scientific medical articles and hundreds of books which have been my regular companions over these decades. I re-read and learned things that I had not encountered for many years. I try to read today's news and editorial comments. I try to be balanced in my core attitudes while suffering from optimism and idealism. I freely confess to being an intellectual gadfly sticking my nose into disciplines remote from my own.

Out of this heady ferment "Next Medicine" emerges. I hope that Granddaddy would be proud.

# Contents

# Foreword

*"Medicine is a science of uncertainty and an art of probability,"* said Sir William Osler, an architect of the Johns Hopkins School of Medicine and its contribution to the 20th century transformation of medicine as a profession, from one often resembling alchemy to one intended to focus on science, the evidence, and the patient. Through his insistence that medical education include ample interaction with patients—e.g. *"He who studies medicine without books sails an uncharted sea, but he who studies medicine without patients does not go to sea at all"*—and his establishment of the post-graduate residency apprenticeship, Osler's firm belief in the centrality of understanding the patient's perspectives, insights, and circumstances is clear. In the face of complexity and individual variation, certainty is rare, and dependence on an informed calculus of likelihood and probability, the requirement. It's about the individual and his or her context.

Walter Bortz describes in an artfully engaging manner how today's medicine has seriously strayed from this basic principle, and it may take *Next Medicine* to get it right. With a mix of biology, history, sociology, demography, economics, and politics—even a little religion—Dr. Bortz reflects on the evolution and nature of medical care today to illustrate the view that not only has the business of medicine distracted the focus from the individual, but it has also deflected attention from the societal—the perspectives, resources, and actions necessary to help us stay healthy—and the personal level of control we can exert in maintaining health.

The first half of the last century was a period of great progress in health and medicine. It was a period in which the professionalism envisioned by Osler began to take hold in the medical community, in which sanitation and food safety measures made cities safer places to live, in which the development of antibiotics and vaccines ushered in impressive gains against infectious disease killers, and in which life expectancy at birth increased from age 49 in 1900 to nearly 70 in 1950. These were gains achieved through a growth in the capacity of public health and a strong partnership between the public health and practicing clinician communities.

But also during this period were sown seeds of more challenging times to come—both in the nature of the prominent diseases and the misplaced confidence in the technologic dimension of medicine. The use of tobacco by men rapidly rose and women began to smoke in greater numbers, lifestyles became more sedentary, a revolution occurred in the quantity and nature of food available, workplaces assumed new hazards, all of which contributed to later rises in chronic disease killers such as heart and lung disease, stroke, cancers, and diabetes.

Simultaneously, encouraged by previous successes against single diseases such as pneumonia, tuberculosis, diphtheria, pertussis, tetanus, and other childhood vaccine-preventable diseases, and fueled by post-war economic growth, the nation's health and medical attention and resources riveted on diagnosis and treatment of the chronic diseases—the most prominent of which became singular foci of the research, medical, commercial, and policy communities.

With attention directed to the construction of new hospitals, the application of new diagnostic and imaging technologies, the drama of an organ transplanted successfully, the resulting professional, economic, and cultural incentives promoted a disproportionately reductionist focus on diseases at the expense of attention to the intersecting elements of their etiologies, consequences, and prevention. Specialization in focus and technology offered a sense of the scientific, but without consideration to Osler's admonition to tend to the full picture, the attendant scientific uncertainty, or the knowledge of the variable issues and probabilities that may pertain to a given patient. Engaging the complex and the personal—not to mention the social and the political— essentially became too time-consuming, running counter to the prevailing incentives.

If one wishes to take a poignantly expressive and crisply informed tour through this half century of rapid change in American medicine—tracing to factors in play three millennia back—there can be no more interesting lens through which to view it than that of a keen observer raised in a medical family molded in the spirit of the physician-citizen who is steward not only of informed treatment of illness, but of understanding engagement of the forces that shape health. That is the tradition and commitment that Walter Bortz brings to us in *Next Medicine*.

Apart from the service provided in a concise and accessible compendium on significant historical milestones in the evolution of health and medicine in society, Dr. Bortz notes that his mission is "to help reclaim medicine's nobility of service to humanity." He leads us on a journey that draws on his own interesting life and experiences to trace the roots of that spirit, identify inflection points, emphasize failures and their sources, and posit remedies—all the while introducing important players who he encourages to speak to us, as they have to him, along the way.

Although certain of the voices he summons are those of philosophers, archeologists, historians, world leaders and scientists offering testament on earlier days, many are contemporary leaders in basic science, economics, politics, ethics, public health, and medicine. And they speak often in unrestrained terms of protest at conditions in health care today, as does Dr. Bortz in listing and elaborating on the prominent symptoms he sees: excessive cost, injustice, harmfulness, corruption, inefficiency, and irrelevance.

While acknowledging the life-saving potential already in hand with many advances in diagnostic, medical and surgical interventions, and many more to come with breakthroughs in genomics, molecular biology, and robotics, he expresses concern at casual overreliance on these approaches. The terms he chooses to describe Current Medicine are unequivocal in the perspectives described, e.g. "technologic imperative", "medical industrial complex", "fragmented", "over-specialized", "disease cartel".

In many ways, *Next Medicine* offers testament to the need for reform of health care akin to that passed in the Patient Protection and Affordable Care Act of 2010, with its intended aim of not only reducing the patchwork and gap-filled nature of health insurance coverage, but of shifting economic incentives to reward care that is more effective and produces healthier outcomes at lower costs, to reduce geographic and social disparities in care, improve the rewards for primary care, and to strengthen preventive services and public health capacity. The fact that many of the provisions seek to produce the information on which to deliver and measure outcome-oriented care reflects a prevalent concern about the issues that Dr. Bortz addresses.

Ultimately, it is more personal than this. For Walter Bortz, Next Medicine is that "which emphasizes self-efficacy and individual responsibility and insists on studying the total organism over time." In an obvious labor of joy and love, he presents a fascinating and compelling review of studies, stories, and personal observations that illuminate and illustrate the notions he emphasizes on the inherent resilience, plasticity, and durability of the body as an integrated system; the power of activity and engagement in maintaining the balance and functionality of the system; and the necessity of realigning the administrative, social and political structures to support this personal empowerment.

While we cannot predict whether the synchronous alignment of these forces will indeed yield the 100 healthy years that Dr. Bortz identifies as our natural endowment, or extend the maximum attainable beyond 130, the basic premise is indisputable that the prevailing allocation of attention and resources in health is woefully misconfigured to capture that potential. And, although the studies available to Dr. Bortz were not yet imagined in Osler's time, it is highly likely that, compared to the state of play in medicine today, Osler would take much greater comfort in the Next Medicine described by Walter Bortz.

J. Michael McGinnis, MD, MPP*
Washington, DC

* Dr. McGinnis is Senior Scholar at the Institute of Medicine of the National Academies in Washington DC. Views expressed are his, and not necessarily those of the Institute of Medicine or the National Academies.

# Preface

*If you would die fagged to death like a crow with the king birds after him, be a schoolmaster.*

*If you would wax thin and savage like a half-fed spider, be a lawyer.*

*If you would go off like an opium eater in love with your starving delusions, be a doctor.*

—*Oliver Wendell Holmes (1)*

I am a physician, but I did not need opium to fall in love with my profession. I embraced medicine passionately. Each of the myriad errands I performed in its service I performed with enthusiasm and idealism. I loved night and emergency room summonses. I volunteered to be on call over the holidays. My decades as a physician have overflowed with thousands of close encounters—office visits, house calls, ICU challenges, laboratory experiments, lectures—and immersion in both professional organizations and aging-related community activities. Each was imbued with the spirit of Oliver Wendell Holmes's advisory.

I was surely a doctor before I was born—the profession was in my umbilical cord blood. My father was a physician and a genuine alpha male, president of his high school class and captain of the undefeated, unscored-upon state football championship team. He attended Harvard College and Harvard Medical School, where he studied with some of the legendary icons of medicine.

I was born in 1930, as Dad's practice was growing, and was named after Dad's older brother Walter, who was for more than 70 years a devoted internist to the gentle people of Greensburg, Pennsylvania, the birthplace of both my parents. Mom and Dad settled into a tiny rowhouse in downtown Philadelphia, and this was home for the first 16 years of my life. The first floor housed Dad's waiting room, office, and examining room, so I was constantly reminded to play softly whenever I practiced the piano. I recall overflow patients waiting on the stairs to the second floor. Dad often wrote off the fee for his services, or accepted payment in some form of barter. I remember boxes of cherries after one patient visit, and still hanging in my home today are three oil paintings by a down-on-his-luck Russian painter, Leonid Gechtoff, who paid Dad the only way he could.

When I was growing up, Dad and Uncle Walter not only took me on house calls, they also recruited me to make hospital rounds. I listened to heartbeats and felt bumps long before I had the slightest idea of what I was doing. In 1947, while I was still in high school, Dad was elected president of the American Medical Association, becoming the youngest president in that organization's 100 years. He had somehow managed to become a premier politician while also working as a solo medical practitioner. To both his new post and his work he brought independence, self-reliance, leadership skills, and humanity. Dad's precocious interest in aging, which he attributed to his worship of my grandfather, was one of the principal sparks that led Ethel Percy Andrus to found the AARP, as legend has it, in our dining room (2,3).

I studied premed at Williams College, where I wrote my honors thesis on atherosclerosis (4). In 1951, I was admitted to the University of Pennsylvania Medical School before the transcripts of my grades were received because, I believe, Dad was a good friend of most of the faculty. I married the daughter of a physician, an all-purpose practitioner in Watertown, Massachusetts, whose driveway was the first one the police would plow whenever a blizzard struck. Many of the town's male babies were named Charles in his honor. He took out my wife's tonsils, and her sister's, on the kitchen table. His accounting system was a drawer in the hall table, stuffed with crumpled five-dollar bills.

Soon after Ruth Anne and I married, we met another major figure in our personal and professional lives. My father's good friend Dr. Nils Paul Larsen was the acknowledged father of modern medicine in Hawaii. Ruth Anne and I wanted to go to Honolulu on our honeymoon. In the summer of 1953,

Dr. Larsen paid me a dollar an hour to review the autopsy records of those who had died in that island's Queen's Hospital. Our subsequent report clearly showed marked racial differences in the incidence of hardening of the arteries among the deceased. Scarcely noticeable in the Japanese and Filipinos, it was moderate in the Chinese and significant in the Hawaiians and Caucasians (5). This led to the observation that the Japanese in Hawaii had intermediate levels of artery hardening—more than in Tokyo but less than in Los Angeles. Their genes had not changed, but their lifestyles had. This central observation was to stimulate the remainder of my career and eventually led to the permanent establishment of the acclaimed Hawaii Heart Study, all of which originated from that honey-moon project.

After earning my MD in 1955, I spent a year as an intern with my father at the Lankenau Hospital, a then-new hospital in suburban Philadelphia. It was the direct product of my father's association with Miss Ethel Pew, one of the principals of the Sun Oil dynasty, who had become captivated by his worldview. She charged him with bringing a vision of the hospital of the future to the draw-ing board. So, just inside the hospital's entrance, he set up the Health Museum, which presented dozens of exhibits on how to stay healthy (6). The research division was consecrated to projects dealing with health rather than disease.

This was a radical concept then, much as it is now. But it is a concept that has informed my work for most of my life. Even at that young age, I grasped the prevailing notion that hospitals are places of suffering. But this is not how it should be. To Hippocrates' injunction that Medicine should strive to cure sometimes, to relieve often, and to comfort always, we should add the require-ment "to educate first." After all, the word "doctor" comes from the Latin "docere," meaning "to teach." Health illiteracy is the greatest killer of all. My early life, spent at my father's side, set a "health first" agenda that has directed the rest of my career and is the central theme of this book.

I began my formal training in internal medicine at Charity Hospital in New Orleans, a virtual MASH unit, and then went on to the University of California in San Francisco for another year as an internal medicine resident, and 2 addi-tional years in a biochemistry lab at UC Berkeley doing research on fat metabo-lism. From Berkeley we gathered up our four kids and went to Munich, where in my third year of postdoctoral fellowship I worked with Professor Feodor "Fitzi" Lynen at the Max Planck Institute for Cellular Chemistry. Fitzi won the Nobel Prize the next year. He honored my work with him in the conclusion to his acceptance speech in Stockholm in 1962 (7).

Finally we returned to Philadelphia, where I joined my father at his hospital. We shared patients, dreams, and speeches. I made hundreds of house calls, but

I also ran a major research program on fat metabolism, supported by NIH grants that were readily forthcoming following my successes in Lynen's laboratory. It was an intense 10 years.

When Dad died at 74 as the result of an accumulation of causes, I was devastated. I could not sleep, eat, or work. I was seriously, clinically depressed. It took three life-altering developments to finally, slowly, heal my grief.

First, I started to run. I had never run before and am a slow, awkward runner, but I knew that running was the finest medicine for depression. I ran the Boston Marathon that year and have run a marathon a year for 40 consecutive years since, including Beijing in 2006, New York, in 2008, and Boston in 2010.

Second, we moved back to San Francisco in 1972, where I had an appointment at Stanford University and the Palo Alto Medical Clinic. Gone was the absolute autonomy of solo practice, but substituting the pay-as-you-go pattern with a regular paycheck more than compensated. Moreover, the rich give-and-take of group practice instilled civility and taught me participatory governance. The group valued and rewarded hard work. The PAMC appointment gave me an affiliation with the renowned Stanford Hospital and Medical School across the street, where I cared for my hospitalized patients and participated in academic activities. With funds donated by several grateful patients, I set up a small 501(c)3 foundation, the Active Living Institute, to fund important research programs and public lectures that have allowed me to get to know such wonderful presenters as Jared Diamond, Art Linkletter, Richard Dawkins, and others.

The third life-shaping change was my immersion in geriatrics. My father had had an early involvement in aging issues; he lectured and wrote about it and encouraged my interest in it (8). I became a geriatric specialist and built a substantial practice as well as launching numerous research projects. I have pursued the science of aging with enthusiasm. I have been a caring steward of thousands of aging patients and have presided at hundreds of deaths. I have involved myself in the organizational aspects of the issue, becoming chairman of every local community aging activity, including the East Palo Alto Senior Center, where, as the only white member of an all-African-American constituency, I served as president.

In 1983, I became president of the American Geriatrics Society, an organization of which my father had been a founding member. Geriatrics is a special case for medicine. Aging is not a disease, so it falls outside the scope of traditional pathologies. There is no cure for the role of time in the aging process. Aging requires its own set of definitions and guidelines. Today's practice of medicine must broaden its view to include the aging continuum in its understanding and reach.

In many ways, I view my current mission—to help reclaim medicine's nobility of service to humanity, the tradition from which my profession originally sprang—as carrying on much of the work that was started by one John Gardner, a man who was, in my view, one of the greatest and most influential Americans of the last 100 years. Gardner was the founder of Common Cause, and as Lyndon Johnson's Secretary of Health and Human Services he was responsible in many ways for Johnson's civil rights initiatives. He also presided over the introduction of Medicare, with which my father and his AMA affiliations were closely involved. Gardner indoctrinated me in his total devotion to the primacy of community in all human affairs.

Finally, I must mention the importance of Norman Cousins to my work. His extraordinary 1976 article in the *New England Journal of Medicine*, "The Anatomy of an Illness," was a marvelous description of his recuperation from a life-threatening illness, an ill-defined immunological disorder that could not be concretely diagnosed (9). It made a huge impression on me, and his published work on medical matters led me to invite him to join me to speak to an AMA meeting in Las Vegas on wellness issues. He and I bonded and became intimate friends during the last 10 years of his life. I cherish the inscriptions he wrote to me in his later books, and a letter from him is among my most prized possessions.

Cousins could captivate listeners for hours with stories of his encounters with such luminaries as Albert Schweitzer, Pope John, Einstein, Roosevelt, Churchill, and countless others. He posed the same question to each of them: "What have you learned in life?" The answers he got ranged from awkward and crude to richly perceptive. In our conversations, he and I agreed that human experience is the most precious resource on earth—yet it is not on anyone's list of recyclable materials. Glass, paper, soda cans, even cow manure get renewed, yet human experience vanishes at its origin.

Why couldn't Uncle Walter and my father have debriefed themselves fully to me before they died? Why can't all of us on our 75th or 90th or 100th birthday go to the town library and record a 15-minute report on "what I have learned"? I shared this thought one day with Nils Nilsson when he was director of the Stanford computer science program. "Have you heard about the deepwell diggers?" Nils asked. These, he said, are people like the famous Red Adair, who are summoned to Kuwait or Galveston or other such locations to put out oil rig fires. A tiny clan of experts, most of these individuals never graduated from college or wrote a book, but they possess critical knowledge on which huge dollars and many lives depend. Recognizing their preciousness and that their knowledge is very perishable, some smart people decided to debrief Red and his colleagues on "What have you learned?" Their unique know-how became a matter of survival.

Along the same theme, the redemptive value of human experience is contained in a small book, *Two Old Women*, by Velma Wallis (10). It is a gentle retelling of an ancient Athabascan legend. In the depth of a cruel Alaskan winter, starvation threatens the tribe, and the chief announces, "The council and I have arrived at a decision. We are going to have to leave the old ones behind." The two old women who are abandoned watch their loved ones trek into the cold night and begin their own death vigil. But their desperation eases as they tend their last ember. They blow on it, and it flares anew. They trap a rabbit and snare a squirrel. One of the women vaguely remembers a fishing hole over the next ridge and around a bend. Miraculously, they find it and catch food from beneath the frozen creek. Their strength returns, life re-emerges.

Meanwhile, the tribe grimly endures. The guilt-ridden chief retraces his steps to bury the old women, only to find them gone. A search party discovers them by the fishing hole, melancholy but full of health and vitality. The old women become the salvation of their tribe. Their experience and knowledge ensure the group's survival.

This perspective is what prompts me to write this book. It is my effort to download the incredible things I have learned. I am fully aware of the extraordinary good luck I have enjoyed. I can count the bad days in my life on a very few fingers. I figure that all of this richness and opportunity only deepen my responsibility to debrief.

I hope that the result, this book, is worthy. Proud to have consecrated my life to the idealism of medicine, this is my "deep-well digger" testament. It also represents my best effort to recapture the first principles of medicine, which Hippocrates identified 2,500 years ago, and to use them to build a new model, one that provides more adequately for humanity's deepest needs than has the medicine of recent memory.

My father called medicine a jealous mistress. I was and continue to be an earnest suitor. Its demands ordained one of the few major sadnesses of my life, as I did not really see my four children grow up. I am spending the rest of my years trying to make up for this dereliction (grandchildren are partially redemptive), but I love my profession and cannot even imagine an alternative life. I was a privileged participant in a Golden Age of medicine that delivered humanity from smallpox and polio. Now, at a time when my profession is under assault from nearly all sides, I lobby for medicine's success. I wallow in its triumphs, but I also sorrow in its inadequacies and its misadventures, its misdirections and its cost.

The past 20 years have generated a rising crescendo of critique as medicine has strayed from its central commitment to personal well-being and has become industrialized. Some of our leaders ask whether medicine has lost its soul. I was originally deaf to such complaints, but now I hear tones that cause me embarrassment and shame, that both anger me and provoke feelings of guilt. This fall from grace happened on my watch. I must be part of the problem. My pride is bruised by this recognition, but apologizing for a broken promise is not productive. Instead I hope to be a part of a solution that may allow medicine to reclaim the high ground.

# Medicine's Mission | 1

One day in 2006, I was in the pit of the lecture hall at Meharry Medical College in Nashville, where I was to speak before a group of second-year medical students on "Successful Aging." Meharry was founded in 1876 and is one of two surviving black medical schools created in the 19th century.

I scanned the faces of my audience of about 200 mostly female would-be doctors and flashed back to when I was a second-year student at the University of Pennsylvania School of Medicine, 50 years before. Eisenhower was president then. Color TV was just emerging. Jackie Robinson was an All-Star. Elizabeth was crowned queen of England. Everest was climbed. DNA was discovered. The civil rights movement was in its early stirrings; the next year, Rosa Parks would refuse to move from the front of the bus.

Who had I been then? Who were these students now? I was an alien in their midst. I was male, they were female. I was old, they were young. I was white, they were black. But I recognized that it was neither gender nor age, geography nor race that separated me from them so much as it was time. The past 50 years have brought enormous changes to medicine. The setting of the medical drama of the 1950s was bucolic, simple, and gentle. There was little external oversight. Physicians of my time were accountable only to our own consciences. Today's medical drama is all skyscrapers and huge corporations.

My career began in the "doctor as god" period that lasted from Hippocrates until Ralph Nader and the rise of consumerism. A culture of questioning authority has displaced the power of the paternalistic physician, as Mark Siegler of the University of Chicago described it in his 1985 article, "The Progression from Physician Paternalism to Patient Autonomy to Bureaucratic Parsimony," published in the *Archives of Internal Medicine* (1). The patient autonomy era was very short-lived, and we have quickly been thrust into the parsimonious administrative era, where what prevails is neither what the physician nor the patient desires, but what some anonymous insurance clerk in Hartford or elsewhere decides shall come to pass.

The Meharry students will learn more about insurance than they will ever want to know. They will meet corporate and administrative people whose jobs were not even a glimmer on the horizon in my day. When I was a med student, doctors were modest in their financial dealings. Good Samaritanism ruled. Today's med students will be thrust into dealings with collection agencies. The medicine of my second-year med school experience was meager, but it was gentle and generous. Today students will enter a thoroughly corporate milieu.

In my view, two main forces have been driving these changes. The first is the knowledge explosion. Knowledge is said to double every 15 years or so. So in the 50 years since I graduated from med school, medical science has acquired eight times more know-how. Our collective ignorance no longer vastly exceeds our collective knowledge. My father recalled that when he entered Harvard Medical School, his dean declared, "Ladies and gentlemen, the next four years will be the greatest intellectual experience of your lives. You will learn all the elements of the human body, its structures and functions, and its defects. Unfortunately half of what we teach you will no longer be true in several years. And further, we don't know which half that is."

Lewis Thomas, another of my real-life heroes, made a similar observation in 1935. Thomas had a distinguished career in academic medicine at Johns Hopkins, Duke, and Yale Medical Schools, and eventually served as President of the Memorial Sloan-Institute. In his 1983 book *The Youngest Science*, he reflected on his memories of his second year at Harvard Medical School: "During the third and fourth years of school we also began to learn something that worried us all. Although it was not much talked about, it gradually dawned on us that we didn't know much that was really useful, that we could do nothing to change the course of the great majority of the diseases which we were so busy analyzing, that medicine, for all its façade as a learned profession was in real life a profoundly ignorant occupation" (2).

In retrospect, medical practice in my day combined a dependence on tradition with a good deal of risk. We kept heart attack victims in bed for 2 weeks after their acute episode, certainly adversely affecting their survival. We treated ulcers with the "Sippy Diet," half milk and half cream, two ounces every hour to "soothe" the stomach, a naïve concoction of no value. My wife Ruth Anne was hospitalized routinely for 10 days after our first baby was born, yet today we know that bed confinement courts all sorts of mischief, chiefly blood clots.

When my grandfather Bortz was stricken with pneumonia, my physician dad and uncle were at his bedside. They were shaken by his struggle to breathe. The first of the sulfa medicines, sulfanilamide, was just being released. Somehow, the doctors Bortz got hold of some of the first samples. They gave it to their father, and for several days he seemed to improve. His fever and his breathing eased. But several days later, his condition worsened again, and he died at age 74 after ailing for a week or two. I remember the grieving that followed. In retrospect, it was not the pneumonia that killed him, but the sulfa medicine. Dad and Uncle Walter were simply unaware that the first sulfa drugs were highly insoluble; they crystallized in the kidney and led to uremia unless the patient was given copious amounts of fluid.

On the other hand, I can also still vividly see the hospital room and the figures around the bed where the 11-year-old son of one of my father's closest friends lay desperately ill with meningitis. The damp, antiseptic air felt darkly ominous. Somehow, Dad had procured some penicillin; it was urgently administered with joyful results. This is an example of the baby steps with which medical progress proceeds, making many missteps along the way.

The second force that has so dramatically driven changes in the practice of medicine is, of course, the money explosion. Not only is today's medicine more knowledgeable, it is also vastly richer. Fifty years ago we spent 4% of our gross national product on health care. In 2010, it approaches 20%, or $2.5 trillion per year. That is $5 billion per day, or $4 million per minute. This is a far cry from the Spartan ledger sheet that existed in my father's day. Medicine is the single largest enterprise in our nation. Instead of the humble cottage industry of the past, the solo practitioner of my era, med students now enter a huge corporate industry. They are sitting on a vast treasure trove of knowledge and money. It should be heaven; but this bonanza comes at an immense price.

Paul Starr, a Princeton professor and the author of the Pulitzer Prize-winning book, *The Social Transformation of American Medicine*, describes the current era as "medicine's fall from sovereignty" (3). Perhaps we in my era were sovereign, but we had limited knowledge and financial resources with which to address our job. With our magnificent new technology—isotopes, MRIs, and more—we can trace single atoms. We know where they are, where they are going, what they are doing. We have a profound understanding of nature and nature's ways that was previously completely hidden from us. But the complexity of this new treasure means that we have to think in entirely new and different ways.

## Defining Medicine's Mission

Despite the huge knowledge and fiscal gulfs that separate the Meharry students' time from mine, we are joined by one unifying element—medicine's mission. Our profession stretches back into prehistory, and has an almost infinite future. Yet I know of no one who has bothered to come up with a rigorous mission statement for medicine. What is its job description? Just what, after all, is medicine supposed to do?

As I search for the first principle(s) from which all else derives, I offer as a terse definition: "Medicine's mission is to assert and assure human potential." In a parallel vein, Norman Cousins ventured that "the physician's role is to help mankind make of itself the most of which it is capable" (4). Put yet another way, the physician's job is not only to cure illness or to fix broken bones, but to serve first as a mirror into which the patient peers to see the reflection of the problem, and secondly as a prism showing not just what is, but what might be. The physician's role transcends that of simple mechanical repair. The human body is infinitely more than a deterministic machine.

Doctors past, present, and future share this common mission. Remember that *docere* means "to teach." What is it that medicine teaches? It teaches us our nature. It is a survival manual—but also more.

Understanding medicine's mission means grappling with the idea of human potential. My personal philosopher is William James, whose pragmatism informs my life and outlook. One of his central axioms is, "We live lives inferior to ourselves" (5). What he is saying is that our human potential is somewhere out there to be explored as we dare. Yet it has not been rigorously addressed. We have not previously had the tools to measure human potential fully, but the past few decades have yielded warehouses full of data on our most intimate details. We know our anatomy and physiology. We are close to being able to answer the Delphic oracle's command, "Know thyself," with, "We do."

Consider, for example, the savant syndrome. The savant has an otherworldly computational ability and is capable of intellectual deeds that are ordinarily unimaginable. And yet we know so little about this syndrome. Examples of extreme performance—whether physical, psychological, creative or intellectual— should serve as benchmarks of the kind of superior lives that we might live. I believe that it is medicine's job to outline our potential with our new ability to define not only how long we can live, but also the central factors that determine that duration. It is impossible to react to James's observation if we do not know what our potential truly is.

Medicine's mission is definable and ongoing, but it also evolves. In 1984, a woman with amyotrophic lateral sclerosis sued the state of New Jersey, asking to be taken off life support. The New Jersey Supreme Court ruled in her favor in that landmark case. In her assenting opinion, Justice Marie Garibaldi wrote, "Matters of fate have become matters of choice" (6). In these terse eight words she described a momentous transition. From a passive acceptance mode, medicine's mission has evolved into an active interventionist philosophy. Before, medicine's nature/nurture interface was random, unknowing fate. But our new enlightenment has altered the interaction, which is now informed by choice. Yet so far it appears that we have chosen a nurture—a health care system—that does not match our nature.

## A Mission Not Accomplished

Medicine's mission statement must take into account that it is a profession. A 1966 book, *Professional Men: The Rise of the Professional Classes in 19th-Century England,* by W. J. Reader, described a profession as an occupation that (1) regulates itself through systematic required training and collegial discipline, (2) is based on technical and specialized knowledge, and (3) has a service rather than a profit orientation enshrined in its code of ethics (7). The famous Hippocratic Oath is an ethical code of conduct.

For medicine, the third item has become a sticking point. Over the past few decades, we have seen hundreds of instances in which financial reward has skewed the Samaritan imperative that is supposed to guide physicians. As a result, the profession has become weakened and ill, and unable to accomplish its mission. I hear my profession groan, and the illness is severe, not a "take two aspirin and call back in the morning" sort of affair. Medicine is a patient with an ailment so serious as to require intensive care, and most assuredly a transplant.

As we anticipate developments in the anxious and crowded waiting room, we overhear the patient's crescendoing cries of distress. In 2002, Mark Schlesinger published a paper in the *Milbank Quarterly* titled "A Loss of Faith: The Source of Reduced Political Legitimacy for the American Medical Profession" (8). In it he cited three large polls conducted from 1965 to 1999. From a high of 80% public support for the medical profession in 1965, the figure had fallen to 40% by 1999. In a 30-year period, American medicine went from perhaps the most trusted to one of the least trusted social institutions.

The general deference traditionally accorded medicine has been undercut by diminished public confidence in its ability to carry out its mission. Medicine suffers not from "mission creep," enlarging on original goals, but from "mission failure."

This general discomfort with the profession has surfaced before—during the Truman, Nixon, and, more recently, the Clinton and Bush administrations. Every survey reflects a near consensus that the situation is bad, medicine's mission is ill defined or not completed.

But just because the situation is intractable does not mean that it is impossible. As my Stanford colleague Paul Romer, and more recently President Obama's chief of staff, Rahm Emanuel, proposed, "A crisis is a terrible thing to waste." Or, as Common Cause founder John Gardner frequently observed, "What we have before us is a glittering opportunity of unrivaled promise, which is disguised as an insoluble problem."

This combination of opportunity and problem requires a revolutionary response. This is something that Thomas Kuhn, the noted historian of science at the University of Chicago, recognized in his 1962 book, *The Structure of Scientific Revolutions* (9). He asserted that the emergence of a new theory is generally preceded by a pronounced professional insecurity, a sense of malfunction, a major malaise. That insecurity is generated by the persistent failure of the puzzles of normal science, or politics, to come out as they should. Failure of existing rules is the prelude to a search for new ones.

Kuhn's tenets fit medicine's present circumstance precisely. What is needed is a rigorous new alternative, a new paradigm, more complete than the former paradigm. Medicine's current paradigm is not cost-effective, fair, safe, honest, efficient, or relevant. It falls far short of fulfilling Medicine's mission of asserting and assuring human potential.

Asserting our potential is not the hard part of the mission. For the first time in human history, we have a clear view of what a whole human life can look like. We know its extent and its content. Our potential stands revealed for the first time, a gift that is worthy of a hundred Nobel Prizes. None of the prior 151 billion of us has known what he or she was capable of. Now we know better the space, span, and pace of our potential, as I will describe in later chapters. The human being is a masterpiece of nature's design. Our near perfection is no random accident or metaphysical gift, but the result of relentless surveillance and engineering by our adaptive capabilities. It includes an extraordinary self-repair capacity. I will argue that 100 healthy, fully functional years is each human's potential. It is impossible to overstate how empowering this knowledge is.

## A New Paradigm: Next Medicine and the Return of Hygeia

The new paradigm is Next Medicine, a rebalancing of disease medicine and health medicine. Two thousand five hundred years ago, the Greeks identified medicine's twin components: Hygeia and Panacea, or health preservation and repair. Of these, Hygeia, the preservation of health, originally held precedence. Today, Panacea, repair, dominates. Panacea's elaborate repair capacities are brilliant, but its toolkit of surgery and pharmacy does not fully ensure that we humans will reach our full potential. Next Medicine welcomes Hygeia back as an important member of the medical family.

Plato noted that life without health is not worth living. This means that creating and maintaining health must be a priority. By embracing repair and cure, and the huge financial rewards inherent therein, medicine has neglected the maintenance and prevention aspects that are the essence of health. Next Medicine is a total recommitment to the precious first principles that the Greeks declared long ago, and brings disease medicine and health medicine together once again. Next Medicine emphasizes self-efficacy and individual responsibility for maintaining health and offers a new conceptual framework for health, the study of the total organism over time.

This conceptual shift from a disease-centric to a health-centric model is undeniably cataclysmic, and the tectonic forces it will set loose are bound to reverberate widely. The practitioners of and investors in Current Medicine will protest mightily and hunker down to protect their territory, just as their counterparts did in the past. Think of Charles Darwin, who wrote in *On the Origin of Species,* "Although I am fully convinced of the truth of the views given in this volume, I by no means expect to convince experienced naturalists, whose minds are stocked with a multitude of facts all viewed during a long course of years, from a point of view directly opposite to mine" (10).

Navigating the shift will take courage, but I am convinced that it is a shift whose time has come. It is a shift that the Meharry students and their generation will have to preside over. Extending nobility and legitimacy to Next Medicine will be a complex task, but it can be done, if the will is there. As John Gardner said, "You who would change social institutions cannot be of short wind."

# Current Medicine | I

# Symptoms

A doctor's first meeting with a new patient typically entails a top-down assessment: "Why are you here? What's wrong? Where does it hurt? What are your symptoms?" The patient we are examining here is medicine itself. Current Medicine, as I call it, is a difficult, complex case. It is bothered not by one chief complaint, but by a whole list of symptoms, each with its own urgency. Each one deserves its own analysis, although there are clear feedback loops between many of them, so that addressing one complaint will surely have the complementary effect of ameliorating others.

These symptoms are, in more or less descending order of recognition:

- Cost
- Injustice
- Harmfulness
- Corruption
- Inefficiency
- Irrelevance

All these symptoms have been, and continue to be, exhaustively scrutinized in the media and elsewhere. Usually, however, each one is treated in isolation, out of the context of the whole. As a doctor viewing a patient, though, I am compelled to analyze them together in a search for clues as to how things got so out of control, and what treatments are suggested.

## Symptom 1: Excessive Cost

The central and most vexing problem for medicine today is cost (1). This symptom dominates all the others. What medicine costs today is a long way from a few generations ago, when a house call cost a dollar a visit plus a dollar per mile (two dollars at night), or when a hospital room ran $6 per night, as it did in 1941.

Our total annual medical costs today are $2.5 trillion. If we divide that by the 300 million of us, we are spending an average of $8,200 per person per year on medical conditions and health insurance. That is a figure that consumes a large percentage of a minimum-wage salary, so if we continue at the current rate, medical expenses will soon consume a minimum-wage earner's entire salary.

Every estimate of future medical costs that I am aware of has been grossly underprojected (giving rise to medical futurist Ian Morrison's cautionary note about "premature extrapolation") (2), so that even today's figures are suspect and the next projection in the table is only a stab in the dark.

The escalation has been likened to a trickle becoming a flood, with health care costs on track to totally dominate the gross domestic product (GDP) within three more generations. Nobel Prize-winning economist Robert Fogel of the University of Chicago observed that for every 1% increase in income there has been an accompanying 1.5% increase in health care costs, clearly a nonsustainable relationship (3).

U.S. medical care expenditures are larger than the total GDP of most nations, including China and France. The *WHO Health Report 2000* (which includes 191 countries) (4) reflects that the United States leads the world in one health care category only: cost. The cost to the average German citizen is $2,830. In the United Kingdom it is $2,000, and in Canada $2,700. If we in the

**Table 2.1**

| Year | Total U.S. Medical Care Cost ($) | %GDP |
|------|----------------------------------|------|
| 1940 | $4.1 billion | 3.9 |
| 1950 | $12.7 billion | 4.6 |
| 1960 | $25.9 billion | 5.2 |
| 1965 | Medicare introduced | |
| 1970 | $69 billion | 7.2 |
| 1980 | $230 billion | 8.8 |
| 1984 | $392.7 billion | 11.0 |
| 2009 | $2.5 trillion | 17.0 |
| 2015 | $4.5 trillion (est.) | |
| 2065 | $100 trillion (est.) | |

United States have enough productive capacity to absorb such sick costs, could we not reallocate these trillions of dollars to other social purposes, such as education and preventive health care?

The distribution of these health care costs is also changing. In 1929, 30% of health care costs were attributable to physicians' fees, 23% to hospital charges, 18% to drugs, 12% to dental, 5% to nurses, 3.4% to nontraditional healers, 3.3% to public health, and 4.4% to miscellany. Recent data for 2006 supplied by the Kaiser Family Foundation reflect a significantly altered distribution: physicians' fees are now down to 21.3%, hospital charges have risen to 30.8%, drugs account for 10.3%, nursing home care accounts for 3.9%, home health care accounts for 2.5%, other personal care (dental etc.) accounts for 12.9%, and other health categories make up 16.3% (insurance overhead, research equipment) (5). Although physicians' fees have declined, it should be noted that it is the physician who is the primary gatekeeper for the other charges, so physicians are certainly in a position to affect many of the other health care costs.

Interestingly, drug costs as a percentage of total costs have decreased in the past 80 years, from 18% to 10.3%. But the current top source of cost, hospital care, would certainly be even higher were it not for the major movement toward outpatient surgery, or surgicenters. The facility fee for my recent 4-hour knee arthroscopy was $11,000. Similarly, major surgical advances using endoscopy have reduced the need for hospital care. The advent of specialized surgical hospitals also contributes to these shifting totals.

Even though physicians' fees have decreased as a share of total medical costs, they are still the second most costly component, and the distribution of those fees shows a range of billing power. According to *The Social Transformation of American Medicine* by Paul Starr, the medical profession is the highest-paid occupation in society and receives a radically disproportionate share of the economic pie (6). Data from AlliedPhysicans.com report that the top physician billers are the invasive cardiologists, who gross more than $900,000 a year, and general surgeons, whose gross income is more than $443,000. Thirty-five percent of primary care physicians make more than $200,000 a year (7).

Let's break down the average American health care cost of $8,200 and see what it tells us about how charges are distributed. Figure 2.1 shows that the average percentage of health care expenditures is totally skewed by the high-enders (8). Thirty percent of the total cost is generated by only 1% of the population, and 50% of the cost is generated by 5% of the population; in this percentile, the average cost of health care is $70,000 per person. Seventy percent of the population consumes only 10% of health care dollars, and 40% of the population consumes zero. This shows us how unevenly distributed the demand for health care is.

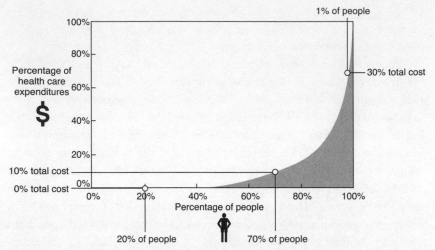

**Figure 2.1** Health care cost continuum: distribution of costs.
Source: Milliman USA Health Cost Guidelines—2010 Claim Probability Distributions.

Let's look further at what skews this distribution. Data from the Agency for Healthcare Research and Quality for hospital discharges in the year 2005 indicate that the most common hospital chart entry is childbirth, at 4 million (9). This is closely followed by 4 million heart-connected diagnoses, 317,000 fractured hips, 616,000 complications related to medical devices or grafts, 401,000 cases of substance abuse, and 101,000 cases of breast cancer. The single costliest diagnosis is newborn distress, which amounts to $114,000 per hospitalization, followed by spinal injuries at $110,000. The median charge for the 200 listed diagnoses is $21,000 per admission (10). The single largest cumulative Medicare expense is related to congestive heart failure: 1.1 million admissions times $28,000 per hospitalization. It is important to think about how many of these diagnoses are actually due to conditions that could be prevented, such as cancers arising from smoking, and how the graph would change if we excluded preventable diagnoses.

Medical cost per productive life is another good measure. What is the measure of a productive life? The American GDP is currently $13 trillion per year. If we divide that by the roughly 225 million citizens between the ages of 15 and 70 (very broadly assumed to be the "productive years"), we get an average yearly per-person productivity of $58,000. If we prorate our $58,000 per year over those 56 years, we get $3.2 million as an average measure of lifetime productivity. If we are then spending $8,200 each of those 56 years, then we have lifetime medical expenses of $459,000, which means that we are spending 15% of our productivity to support our medical needs. Is this appropriate? I say it is not.

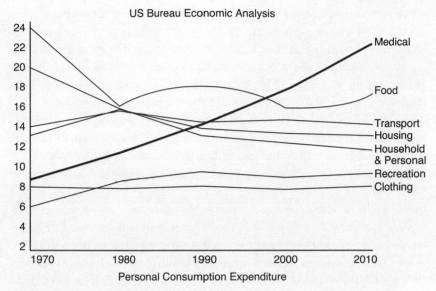

**Figure 2.2** Distribution of expenses.
Source: US Health Economy Analysis 2001.

Clearly, any relevant analysis has to take other things into consideration. What other life activities do we spend money on? Food, housing, clothing, transportation, education, and recreation, among others (Fig. 2.2) (11). In 1960, 17.5% of personal income was spent on food, 5.2% on health care. Now, we spend 9.9% of household income for food and 17% on health care. In a 2004 article in *Health Affairs*, "US Health Care Spending in an International Context" (12) Uwe Reinhardt asks,

> How serious a problem is the alleged economic burden of
> health spending on the US standard of living? Is the medical
> spending as a whole worth it? Should there be alarm about
> the possible reduction in availability of other services?
> In 1970, medical care represented less than one tenth of US
> personal consumption spending, the fifth largest component
> after food, housing, transportation and household opera-
> tion. In that year Americans spent roughly the same portion
> of their personal consumption on clothing as they did on
> medical care. Since then, however, medical care has
> increased steadily in its share of personal consumption.
> The only other major categories of growth since 1970 are
> recreation and personal business expenses.

Reinhardt is notably conservative in his overall judgment as to how much is too much to spend on medical care. Similarly, Harvard's David Cutler is untroubled by the possibility that the United States may spend 20% to 30% of its GDP on health-related expenses, arguing that the more we spend on health, the greater our productivity will be (13). But Ezekiel Emanuel and Victor Fuchs challenge this in a March 2008 article in the *Journal of the American Medical Association* (*JAMA*) (14). There is evidence, they say, that these costs are starting to affect life quality issues. The reason the average hourly wage of workers has been flat since 1982 is that the medical cost escalation has eaten up all of any apparent salary increases, as health insurance premiums have gone up 300% in the past 30 years. In other words, employers are shifting health care charges to the worker's paycheck. General Motors supposedly spends more on medical care than on steel, which has led Warren Buffett to observe that GM is actually a health and benefit company with a car company attached to it (15).

Similarly, as state budgets are stressed by health care costs, states are cutting education appropriations. A 2004 Rockefeller Institute of Government study stated: "The program areas that were most affected by state budget difficulties in 2004 were public higher education. On average, states projected spending 4.5% less on higher education in fiscal 2004 than fiscal year 2003, and raised tuitions and fees by almost 14%" (16). The California Teachers Association buys lots of air time to complain about state education budget cuts; perhaps they should lobby for a healthier state instead (17).

One of the great drivers of cost, of course, is the drug companies' interest in setting new norms and redefining what constitutes a disease. Today, Big Pharma markets diseases, not drugs. It reminds of the late, great comedian Victor Borge, who had a routine concerning his uncle, who became despondent when he discovered a treatment for which no disorder existed.

Then there is the matter of education and health. This was addressed by a study published in the *American Journal of Public Health* in 2007, which showed that what we would save on health care by providing everyone with a college-level education would be eight times what we saved through the use of new drugs and devices developed between 1996 and 2002 (18). Another study, from the New School University in New York, projected that a 5% increase in college enrollment would save $17.1 billion in health care costs. One of my major arguments is that health illiteracy kills more people than all diseases put together.

Since medical expense is so much greater in the United States than in other countries, there is a certain logic to the suggestion that we simply go abroad for treatment when we fall ill. Good idea! There are already a number of groups, such as the Illinois-based company Medretreat, that are promoting this sort of "medical tourism" (19). You can have heart surgery in New Delhi for $15,000, whereas the same procedure costs $85,000 in New York City. We see similar price differences in specialty clinics in Bangkok, São Paulo, and Mexico, to name a few other countries. Many observers are concerned that our higher medical expenses will put us at a competitive disadvantage internationally.

But wait, you say: doesn't the United States have the highest GDP in the world despite its high medical care burden? What if we inverted that argument and said that the United States has the highest GDP *because* it has the largest medical-industrial complex? Based on that reasoning, it should follow that we are rich because we are so sick. This is clearly perverse. Get sick, get rich? Mark McClellan, past director of Medicare, uses the example of an uncomplicated appendectomy in a community hospital. The bill for this procedure might be $6,000. If, however, any complications arise, the bill could easily reach $300,000 (20). Which outcome is better for the GDP, and which would we prefer?

I like to tell the story of a small rural town that became the site of a huge new hospital complex because of the many severe car accidents that occurred at a dangerous mountain curve on its outskirts. The town prospered from the bounty the many injuries brought it. Then a child asked, "Why don't you just put up a guard rail?" My point is similar: Why don't we save a lot of misery and money by embracing prevention?

All these numbers are not abstract economists' figures. They strike at home, directly at our loved ones, friends, and neighbors. Health insurance costs are rising four times faster than a worker's earnings (21). In the past 7 years, out-of-pocket expenses for medical care rose 115%. More than half of Americans say that they are worried about having to pay more for their health care; 42% say they are very worried. Eighty percent of Americans say that they are dissatisfied with high national health care costs and 60% are very dissatisfied. One in four Americans say they have had a problem paying for health care in the past year, and many report delaying medical care because of the expense. A recent study by Elizabeth Warren of Harvard University Law School found that the average debt for persons filing for bankruptcy was $12,000, 50% of which was all or partly due to medical expenses (22). Every 30 seconds in the United States someone files for bankruptcy in the aftermath of a serious health problem. A survey of Iowa consumers found that 86% said that they cut back on how much they save so that they could pay their medical costs, and that they have also had to cut back on food and heating expenses (23). Estimates are that older couples will need close to $300,000 in savings to pay for their anticipated medical coverage.

## Symptom 2: Inequity

"Of all the forms of inequality and injustice," Martin Luther King Jr. once said, "health care is the most shocking and inhumane" (24). Today, the unequal way in which medical care is distributed in this country does indeed strongly imply a pervasive injustice. Archives full of data certify that health care is unevenly distributed based on age, sex, locale, income, education, and ethnicity.

We are born equal, but made unequal by forces often outside our control. This is not what Plato had in mind when he noted in *The Republic* that ensuring equality to all citizens is a prime responsibility of the *polis*, the body politic. The medical profession, as one of the central elements of a democratic society, must commit itself to the pursuit of equality and justice.

Variation in life expectancy is a handy index of inequality. There are many contributing factors to our unequal lifetimes, including wealth and socioeconomic status, ethnicity, health literacy, and geography.

Differences in access to proper nutrition have explained most of humankind's unequal survival to date. But now, access to medical care, insurance coverage, and intensive care unit (ICU) availability are also potential contributors to shorter lives. These factors are not biological, but political.

Of these factors, socioeconomic status is the most determinative. A major report from the World Health Organization addresses the strong association between poverty and physical health (25). It asserts that rising income accounts for three quarters of the increase in life expectancy over the past half-century. Clearly, therefore, improving the economic well-being of the poor is a precondition for better health. The overall health of a country's population in turn permits that country's economic development. Health and wealth are thus intertwined: Call it healthwealth. A broad 2008 survey of the world's nations indicates that the 55 countries with a gross national product of less than $1,000 per person per year and the 100 nations with gross incomes below $2,000 per person per year exhibit markedly lower life expectancy (26). The relationship between life expectancy and income is less clear in countries with GDPs of more than $2,000 per person per year (the United States' is $42,000 per person per year). If we map the United States by socioeconomic status, we see a close coincidence between those states, and even those neighborhoods, with a higher number of "poor" and diminished life quality and expectancy. Hawaii has the nation's highest average life expectancy: 79.8 years. The District of Columbia lags behind at 72.6 years. If we take ethnicity into consideration, the differences are even greater. Asian Americans live to an average age of 85, American Indians to 58.

Once again, are these inequalities due to biology or to politics (27)? As recently as 2000, the mortality rate of blacks was 31% higher than that of whites. A 2002 Institute of Medicine study called "Unequal Treatment: Confronting Racial and Ethnic Disparities in Health" pointed to great disparities between the races in the cost of diagnostic and therapeutic procedures. (28) The NIH's Center for Population Health and Health Disparities catalogs the many differences: The death rate due to asthma is five times higher among blacks than among whites. Nearly twice as many blacks as whites suffer from hypertension, and nearly four times as many from diabetes. Minorities use the emergency department for primary care much more than whites.

The overall incidence of cancer in white America is 477 per 100,000, while it is 512 for blacks and 350 for Hispanics, with corresponding death rates of 191, 239, and 129 respectively. The breast cancer rate is 133 for whites, 118 for blacks, and 80 for Hispanics, but the respective death rates are 25, 34, and 16. Similarly, data on prostate cancer reveal incident rates of 161, 256, and 141 for whites, blacks, and Hispanics, respectively, with death rates of 26, 62, and 21.

Surely these geographical and ethnic inequalities are due primarily to matters of money. People with health insurance live longer, whoever or wherever they are. Access to good health care contributes markedly to survival. It has been calculated that lack of health insurance can account for 20,000 deaths each year. About 200,000 people die yearly without having seen a doctor in the previous year, which testifies to the critical role that insurance plays in health outcomes (29).

Yet the story is even more complicated. I challenge the idea that there is a direct causal relationship between insurance and health outcomes, and I am convinced that adopting a universal health insurance policy, as many advocate, will by itself contribute only marginally to Americans' health. I base this opinion largely on Britain's ongoing Whitehall study, begun in 1996 (30). Since all British citizens have access to the National Health Service, lack of insurance coverage cannot be the reason for differences in health outcomes. Yet an examination of the health statistics of the British civil service reveals substantial differences in such outcomes and in longevity. Dr. Michael Marmot, a professor of epidemiology at University College in London, suggests that this is due to more subtle differences in socioeconomic status (31).

The work of Stanford's Dr. Robert Sapolsky, who maintains his own personal colony of baboons in Kenya, is instructive here. Sapolsky pursues detailed inquiries into the biological differences between the various members of his clan and compares them with the social structure of his group. He finds distinctive biological markers of the hierarchical rankings, complete with endocrine and nervous system function (32). His work is elaborated by Bruce McEwen, whose interest in what is called allostatic load is the human equivalent of Sapolsky's baboon work (33). What both seek is a deeper understanding of how social rank—separate from money, race, or geography—affects how an organism reacts to the nonspecific stresses of life. Their work suggests that it is not money or the other correlates of health that are ultimately determinative, but rather where one ranks in the social hierarchy.

This harks back to the past work of the late Curt Richter at Johns Hopkins (34) and of psychologist Martin Seligman today (35). Both emphasized the term "locus of control" as the critical link between income and health. If people feel that they have little control over their health and their access to health care, then they are less likely to look for solutions to their health problems.

Yet another source of inequality and injustice is the lack of health education and the pervasiveness of health illiteracy in this country. My personal experience working in several Samaritan Clinics, a small group of free medical clinics near Stanford that largely serve Hispanics, points this out to me. At these clinics, language barriers make communication difficult. Care providers do not understand the culture. My patients with diabetes often have no clue about their disease. Many visit me and the clinic solely to get some sample drugs. The results are predictably abysmal. It has been observed that health illiteracy, for which the medical profession shares a major responsibility, causes more deaths than cancer, diabetes, or any other major killer.

Our patchwork insurance non-system is flagrantly inadequate, and health care reform as envisioned by most politicians will not remedy this. How can a nation with spectacular technological apparatus available for some still lag in infant mortality statistics? How can Cubans have longer life expectancy than we do? Medicine at its best is a moral as well as scientific enterprise, and to enjoy such acclaim for our technology while languishing miserably in the social context is unacceptable. The underinsured are not Skid Row reprobates, but people who are often indistinguishable from the rest of us. Our medical system is unjust because it is saturated with all of these inequalities and more.

More than 200 years ago, Thomas Jefferson declared that all humans are born equal. We are made of the same stuff and operate according to the same fundamental biochemical laws. All 6 billion of us share a virtually identical gene portrait, so Jefferson was more right than he knew. We are all born quite equal. Yet our biology shows increasing inequality as we move through life. A recent report in the *Proceedings of the National Academy of Sciences* showed that the genotype (the entire group of genes held in each cell) of identical twins is a mirror image at birth (36). But as the decades pass, differences arise. This indicates that our biology confers near equality at birth, but something happens afterward. One of the things that happens is clearly political: access to health care becomes unequal, and therefore unjust. Our diagnosis of injustice must include a closer examination of the need for health insurance.

Benjamin Franklin spoke of the value of insurance in sharing the risk of unexpected fires (37). It is clear that our national risk of health care disasters is so high that it must be shared. Harvard bioethicist Norman Daniels argues for universal coverage on the basis of distributive justice (38). Distributive justice aims to make a society's distribution of resources fairer, to get better results and outcomes (as opposed to procedural justice, which focuses on administering laws, fair and unfair alike). Daniels says that good health allows people to fulfill their potential, and that it is everyone's responsibility to see that all participate in making this possible. His book *Just Health Care* is a call to guarantee that all citizens (39) are provided the opportunity to participate fully in every aspect of society.

The glaring disparity in health outcomes in America would be partially but still incompletely addressed if we were all to have insurance. Health insurance is not just a good idea; it is imperative. The United States is the only advanced country in the world without an insurance program for all its citizens. Various estimates place our totally uninsured number at 40 million, with another 40 to 70 million underinsured. The Rand Corporation has produced studies indicating that many people fail to pursue recommended therapies and preventive efforts because they lack health insurance (40).

I am convinced that if we are to establish a medical system that fulfills its basic mission, then we must have universal health care coverage. If the medical profession is to deserve its position as one of the central struts of our democracy, it must take a leading role in helping to establish this universal coverage. The majority of medical students and academic physicians support the present administration's push for an insurance plan for all, with no exclusions.

## Symptom 3: Harmfulness

In 1930, Arthur Bloomfield, a distinguished professor of medicine at Stanford, observed, "There are some patients whom we cannot help. There are none whom we cannot harm" (41).

It is a grand irony that one of the largest threats to health in our country is the medical system itself (42). Ralph Nader claims that the U.S. health care system is the single largest preventable cause of death in America (43).

There is a deep historical connection between medicine and harmfulness. Alexander the Great's last words were supposedly, "I'm dying from too many doctors." George Washington was bled to death in a well-intentioned effort to treat his sore throat (44). These historical embarrassments to doctors notwithstanding, tattooed on the frontal lobes of entering medical students is the sacred reminder: first do no harm, *primum non nocere*. This dictum was superfluous for 2,000 years, because although doctors had no effective treatments for most conditions, their mischief along the way was generally limited to isolated opportunities to mistreat.

The past 50 years have changed all this: physicians now have warehouses full of lethal diagnostic and therapeutic weapons to attack our patients with. The archives are replete with well-intended drugs that turned out to be disasters, including thalidomide, chloramphenicol (Chloromycetin), fenfluramine/phentermine (Fen-Phen), and rofecoxib (Vioxx), which have become infamous for their side effects. Even well-intentioned therapies such as hormone replacement therapy turn out, after years, to be doing more harm than good.

The blizzard of new technology is a growing threat. Dr. George Lundberg, former editor of *JAMA*, feels that new enthusiasm for fancy instruments represents "a vast cultural delusion" (45). Further, a recent survey published in *Health Affairs* in 2005 indicates that institutions that feature a great deal of elegant equipment are commensurately deficient in comfort care (46). Machines do not care how you feel, but they pay. The instances of wrong legs being amputated, wrong breasts removed, babies switched, mismatched blood, doubled doses of dangerous drugs, failure to note past allergies, and so on are innumerable.

The elevated risk in medicine is epitomized by ICUs, which have mushroomed in the past 50 years (47). Not coincidentally, they are one of the biggest profit centers for a hospital. The ICU is a venue of high-wire acts in which the chance of a fall is exaggerated by the elevated risk of the patients. Their care is complex, and each layer of complexity presents a new opportunity for misadventure. The risk of a stay in the ICU has been compared to that of coal miners or high-rise construction workers or worse. A study published in *Critical Care Medicine* in 1995 indicated that the average ICU patient experiences 1.7 errors each day, half of which could be termed "critical." Virtually every body orifice has a tube of some sort inserted to administer therapy or to sample body fluids.

Of course, harm can come not just from new drugs and technology, but from doctors themselves. *Iatrogenesis* is the formal term for doctor-generated harm. It comes in two principal varieties: harm associated with surgery and harm associated with prescribed drug treatments. The Institute of Medicine report "To Err Is Human" has spurred a heated response (48).

It is estimated that in the United States, somewhere in the range of 200,000 deaths and 2 million hospitalizations each year are due to iatrogenic misadventure.

That is the equivalent of three packed 747s crashing every day, or three times the total Vietnam casualty list. James James, in his *American Journal of Public Health* article "Impacts of the Medical Malpractice Slowdown in Los Angeles County: January 1976," observed that a few years ago, when doctors went on strike in Los Angeles, the death rate actually went down (49). Many suggest that medicine might look to other industries, such as the aviation industry, to learn their key safety principles, including continued training, emphasis on improved communication, and provision of technical information. In an ideal world, we could make a business case for safety, but the medical-industrial complex is not organized in a fashion that allows for systematic review. That should be possible, however.

A *New York Times Magazine* article on December 14, 2008, described the work of Jerry and Monique Sternin, who run a medical management company and have been working with hospitals nationwide, using a problem-solving approach known as "positive deviance," or PD. These PD programs identify people who have developed coping strategies that work, deviating positively from ineffective standard strategies (50). One PD instance: Jasper Palmer, an orderly at Albert Einstein Medical College in Philadelphia, stuffed harmful, infection-laden hospital gowns into his latex gloves as he was cleaning, creating a safer method for gown disposal. His actions were considered eccentric until someone asked for a systematic review of harm-reducing practices. Now the "Palmer method" is catching on, making patients safer.

Reducing medical harmfulness continues to be a goal, but charges of inattention and incompetence have created a siege mentality within the profession, leading to underreporting of errors and self-protectiveness. One source of slow improvement has been tacitly granting immunity to physicians for owning up to their errors.

Hospitals themselves are a source of harm. Twenty years ago, I was part of a small planning group for a study looking at the functional status of patients who entered, were treated, and were discharged from Stanford University Hospital. Calvin Hirsch, the author of a subsequent paper, noted that many patients were in worse shape when they went home than when they had arrived (51).

My father used to tell the story of a gentle old man who had been in the hospital for more than a week and had resisted all earnest efforts to diagnose his illness. One morning, as my father was leading his medical group on rounds, the fellow addressed him. "Dr. Bortz," he said, "I want you to know, I really appreciate all you're doing to help me, but won't you let me go home for a few days to rest up, and I will be glad to come back and let you work on me some more."

We need a new Sherlock Holmes to expose all the medical errors that have gone unaddressed since medicine became such a hazardous profession. Enter Boston pediatrician Donald Berwick (52). He is a genuine medical hero. In 1999, his wife was stricken by a bizarre illness affecting her spinal cord. She was hospitalized six times in the next 7 months at three of the finest medical centers in the country. Diagnosis and treatment options eluded corps of medical experts. A doctor's wife inevitably receives extra attention (trade secret). Berwick watched and waited and was horrified by the errors he observed being made in his wife's case. No day passed without a new mistake.

Fortunately, his wife's illness passed and she recovered to walk again, but Berwick retained the memory of her bumpy course. He had already been committed to the need for a system that would assess medical performance, but his bedside vigils surely increased his sense of urgency. In 2004, he took the bull by the horns and, with the Health Care Improvement Institute, organized a campaign called "100,000 Lives" (53). The goal was to redress 100,000 avoidable hospital deaths in one year. Which leg to amputate? Which heart attack victim receives aspirin? Which hand-washing protocol is called for? Berwick enlisted 3,100 hospitals and set six precise targets. The early results, still incomplete, indicate that he exceeded the ambitious target; an initial totaling projected that somewhere in the range of 120,000 lives were saved by his simple initiatives.

I find this result monumental, and extremely hopeful for our profession. Everything was done voluntarily, with extensive educational and collaborative effort. It seems obvious that it should be replicated nationwide. This sort of effort is, in effect, a vaccine against physician error, and shows that medicine's harmfulness is not so intractable a symptom as it may at first appear to be.

President Obama, recognizing Berwick's outstanding contributions, on April 19, 2010, nominated him to lead the Centers for Medicare and Medicaid. When confirmed we will have new excellence in a pivotal post that requires guts and smarts.

## Symptom 4: Corruption

When I was president of the American Geriatrics Society and responsible for arranging the program for our annual meeting, I sought and received several thousand dollars from major drug companies, whose generosity we accordingly acknowledged in the program. Following my presidential year, the Pfizer company invited me and 30 presidents of other major medical societies to a series of Presidential Forums. These were swanky affairs held at major resorts and featuring celebrity lecturers. I met Richard Gephardt, then a member of Congress, and former British prime minister Edward Heath, among others. I particularly recall a fascinating dinner conversation in Orlando with State Department ambassador at large Philip Habib, who brought me up to date on conditions around the Gulf of Hormuz. All this was courtesy of our friendly drug company colleagues. But drugs were never mentioned at the meeting. In my various early relationships with the drug-makers, I never felt any sense of guile or undue influence. I welcomed each encounter, particularly with the drug representatives who called to tell me about new products or new information, because they were invariably attractive young women.

In our second-year pharmacology course in medical school, we were taught the ancient and arcane ways of writing prescriptions with common ingredients—so many grams of this, so many drops of that. The neighborhood druggist would, in turn, mix and package them. The relationship between patient, physician, and pharmacist was friendly and professional.

That all seems so long ago. The world was vastly simpler and more transparent then. Physicians and pharmaceutical companies existed specifically to serve the patient. Since then, things have changed dramatically. Those simple days have become a remote memory, as the basic trust between the various parts of the medical system has succumbed to the corporate obsession with profits. The pens and textbooks and sponsored lectureships of my youth have morphed into huge organized influence-mongering that pervades the medical profession. The kingpins of the syndicates are the drug lords and medical-device inventors who respond not to the patient or to the physician, but solely to the stockholder, who, with enough new cash in the till, will turn around and reward the lords and inventors with obscene perks.

Dr. Jerome Kassirer, esteemed past editor of the *New England Journal of Medicine,* wrote an incriminating book called *On the Take* in which he casts a wide net of accusations, sparing no one—professors of medicine, deans of medical schools, officials at the NIH (54). Corruption is possible, and exists, at every level of the medical hierarchy. Kassirer details how the hallowed halls of medical academia have become contaminated by the huge monies involved. Even the sternest review processes are susceptible to compromise when enough money is involved. He relates how the respected medical journal *Annals of Internal Medicine* lost 40% of its advertising revenue after it published a paper that reflected adversely on Big Pharma's marketing strategies (55). The drug companies have huge budgets, which they use to seduce and corrupt young physicians who are eminently at risk because of medical school debts and budding families. The physician's conscience is constantly challenged by the temptations that Big Pharma and big technology offer.

As Kassirer notes, it is not just the drug companies who have brought an element of corruption into the modern medical system. "Doctors are incredibly, horribly responsive to incentives," wrote Harvard's Robert Cutler in *Health Affairs* (17). Professional avarice is everywhere in medicine. In 1990, then-California congressman Pete Stark reacted, promising, "I'll be back with some legislation that will weed out the greedy bastards" (56). No longer are excursions into the netherworld of shadow medicine innocent and harmless and cheap. With the powerful new and expensive technology available, the bad actors are free to scavenge more aggressively, and more dangerously.

Particularly nefarious, as Kassirer shows, is how our "best practices" (using the best current scientific and medical evidence to determine care and treatments) are determined by experts with clear conflicts of interest. Where do we turn when the Bible is written by hired hands? Even the FDA, the authority on which drugs and tools are dangerous and which are valuable, has been penetrated by agents of the drug and medical-device cartels. One of medicine's principal safeguards are the numerous specialty societies that collect and evaluate the data that guide our daily duties. Kassirer notes how many of these prestigious societies are at risk because of one form or another of drug-house subsidies. He fingers cardiology, psychiatry, gastroenterology, urology, oncology, and other main specialties for having discovered ways to hide the fact that they are compromised.

The case of the painkiller Vioxx shows just how tangled the web of corruption and the conflicts of interest have become. The December 12, 2005, *New York Times* article "Ties to Industry Cloud a Clinic's Reputation," along with Paul Krugman's December 16, 2005, *New York Times* piece, "Increasing Corruption in the U.S. Medical and Pharmaceutical Sectors," told the unhappy story of how industry giant Merck obscured the dangers of Vioxx (57,58). A prominent article supporting the drug's safety had appeared in the *New England Journal of Medicine*, but a deeper inquiry revealed that the authors of that Merck-supported research had deleted the unfavorable results. The drug was eventually withdrawn in September 2004 (59).

In December 2005, Dr. Eric Topol was a senior member of the Cleveland Clinic staff, chief of its cardiology unit, and instrumental in the founding of its medical school. Topol had fingered Vioxx as a danger for years and was intimately involved in the disclosures regarding it. He sat on the Cleveland Clinic's conflict-of-interest committee. As such, he was aware that his clinic, in an effort to increase its bottom line, had created a venture capital fund, Foundation Medical Partners. This fund provided money for the development of several products that were in early use with patients at the clinic. One of the spin-off companies, Atricure, manufactured a radiofrequency device used to ablate trouble spots in the heart that are responsible for arrhythmias. Topol's oversight responsibilities created added sensitivity to any ethical breaches. These facts are contained in a December 15, 2005, *Wall Street Journal* article by David Armstrong. 1,247 patients had undergone treatment with this device without being informed that the Cleveland Clinic owned the company whose product had been prescribed for them (60). Other institutions in the Cleveland area also use the device under the direction of a clinic affiliate who receives a $2,000-a-month consulting fee. Central to this connection is Dr. Toby Cosgrove, CEO of the Cleveland Clinic, who until March 2005 had sat on the Atricure board and invested personally in the company. A conflict-of-interest survey forced Cosgrove to step down from the Atricure board. Armstrong reported that four patients treated with the device had died, but when interviewed, Cosgrove had indicated that he was unaware of these deaths. When Dr. Topol's contract came up for renewal at the Clinic, he was put on a form of probation as a reprimand for his whistle-blowing tendency. Topol resigned from the clinic and joined the Western Reserve Medical Center.

Malachi Mixon was the chairman of the Cleveland Clinic Board of Trustees and a former classmate of Raymond Gilmartin, Merck's CEO. They deny any inappropriate conversations about the Vioxx mess. Mixon was also the CEO of Invacare, a health care supply company on whose board sat Bernadine Healy, former head of the NIH and the Red Cross, whose husband had been Cosgrove's predecessor at the Cleveland Clinic. All these interconnections prove nothing, of course, but trust is a central feature of the medical compact. Anything that casts doubt on that trust is troubling.

Medical corruption is particularly evil when it gets into the big business of research grants and drug approvals. Billions of dollars depend on the integrity of those conducting scientific trials and investigations. When that integrity falters, the whole system is affected.

Marcia Angell, respected past editor of the *New England Journal of Medicine*, published a piece in the January 15, 2009, issue of the *New York Review of Books*, "Drug Companies and Doctors: a Story of Corruption" (61). In the article she drew attention to the fact that Senator Charles Grassley, ranking Republican on the Senate Finance Committee, was searching for evidence of inappropriate financial ties between academic physicians, among them professors of psychiatry at Harvard, Stanford, and Emory, and the pharmaceutical industry. One received $1.6 million in consulting and speaking fees between 2000 and 2007. Another held $6 million worth of a psychoactive drug stock, which he trumpeted. Another failed to report $500,000 in income from a company whose drugs he promoted during professional talks.

Angell estimates that U.S. drug companies are spending tens of billions of dollars to influence what physicians prescribe. She says that two thirds of academic medical centers have equity interest in companies that sponsor research within their walls. Two thirds of the directors of medical departments receive departmental income from drug companies. Three fifths receive personal income. Angell considers the medical profession to be more reprehensible than the drug companies, which can at least claim responsibility to their stockholders as an excuse for their shoddy behavior. The professors have no such excuse. Institutions have conflict-of-interest guidelines, but these are only loosely enforced.

In today's medicine, there are big-time hucksters and there are petty hucksters. There is major league malpractice and minor league malpractice. In the latter category are those ubiquitous cases of over-prescribing, over-diagnosing, and over-treating. There is always one more test to order and one more treatment to deliver, all with a rationale behind it, but distorted by the reality that each added measure generates a charge: Am I ordering this cardiogram because it is *really* necessary or because I will receive a fee for it? One of the clear areas of conflict concerns doctor-owned laboratories. These facilities are particularly prone to overuse and are responsible for as much as 44% of excessive charges. Numerous judgments have been rendered against their owners.

Insurance fraud is also big business. An entire industry has sprung up to teach clerks how to "upgrade the diagnostic categories" so that they qualify for higher reimbursement. Such "upcoding" is charging for a more complex service than the one that was actually performed. Billing for services not even rendered is an extreme form of upcoding, and may be more prevalent than anyone knows. Another kind of fraud is physicians charging insured patients more than uninsured ones. And just when you would think you had heard every possible scheme for plundering the medical treasury, an article in the July 2008 *New York Times* reported that congressional investigators had just discovered that Medicare had been bilked of tens of millions of dollars by the illegal use of identification numbers of doctors who had died years ago (62). According to the article, from 2000 to 2007 Medicare paid 478,500 claims containing identification numbers assigned to dead physicians. The amount of money involved is estimated to be between $60 million and $92 million, and in many of these cases the physicians had been dead for more than 10 years. One case involved 10,000 claims totaling $479,000 from 2000 to 2007, even though the doctor in question had died in 1990. These scam artists were treating Medicare like an ATM, drawing out money with little fear of being caught. The U.S. Government Accountability Office (GAO) has estimated that as much as $1 of every $7 spent on Medicare is lost to fraud and insurance abuse (63).

Beyond that, there is more general corruption in the insurance industry. United Health Group, the nation's largest health insurer, was among at least 200 companies that came under scrutiny in 2004 for their backdating practices (illegally changing the date on a claim or stock option to benefit the company/executives). So far, 90 executives have lost their jobs and more than 400 lawsuits have been filed against more than 100 of these companies. Among those trapped was William Maguire, who was forced out as chairman and CEO of United Health in October 2006 after an independent law firm found that his options had been backdated in a fraudulent options scheme, much as in the Enron Corp. scandal. Maguire was forced to relinquish $600 million, while current CEO Stephen Hensley surrendered $190 million (63). Nonetheless, Maguire was allowed to keep $800 million in stock options. One analyst observed that while Maguire's surviving wealth may stick in some people's craw, he did lead the company, for all its flaws, to a significant increase in value for its shareholders from 1988 through 2006, and therefore is entitled to retain some of the benefit for his efforts. Maybe if I were a stockholder, I could feel some generosity toward him, but as a taxpayer I am furious. Meanwhile, millions cannot afford health insurance.

Just as big a business as insurance fraud are unnecessary surgeries (64). As far back as 1974, a congressional inquiry discovered that 2.4 million unnecessary surgeries had been performed the previous year, costing $4 billion and resulting in 12,000 deaths. Uteri, tonsils, appendices, and backs were particularly at risk. By 2004, the Rand Corporation was estimating that 30% of the surgeries performed annually, or about 6 million, representing $19 billion, are unnecessary. The introduction of the first coronary artery bypass in 1968 raised the ante. By 1980, 115,000 of these were being performed; by 1990, there were 230,000, at a cost of $6 billion. A Rand survey described in a 1995 article indicated that 38% of the bypass operations were unneeded (65). When the equivocal category (neither clearly indicated nor contraindicated) is included, the percentage goes up to 64%. The percentage depended heavily on geography.

In 2002, alerted by a courageous practitioner who noted bizarre results with some of his referred patients and who subsequently endured a great deal of harassment as the result of his whistle-blowing, federal agents began an intensive investigation of the Redding, California, Tenet Healthcare Hospital and the practices of Drs. Chae Hyun Moon and Fidel Realyvasquez. They seized hospital records and had them reviewed by outside heart specialists. In 27 years at Redding, Moon had catheterized 35,000 patients, sometimes a dozen per day. At their peak, Moon and Realyvasquez performed nearly 800 open-heart operations in 1 year. In 2001–02, Moon billed Medicare $4 million. The outside medical experts concluded that between one quarter and one half of the patients had been treated inappropriately. Justice Department documents stated that at least 167 patients had died. In 1998, the Redding Medical Center had decided to expand its cardiac laboratories with a five-story addition, and quickly earned $50 million in pre-tax profit.

As a result of the investigation, Tenet agreed to pay $54 million to settle fraud charges, and the company eventually paid $395 million in restitution to 769 patients. Overall, Tenet ended up paying the federal government more than $900 million to settle charges. In 2003, Dr. Moon voluntarily suspended his practice and he and Dr. Realyvasquez agreed to pay $1.4 million each in fines to avoid criminal prosecution. Neither doctor has ever admitted any wrongdoing. In retrospect, lack of oversight was the major institutional failing.

Today, more than 2 million Americans undergo a heart catheterization, and 1.2 million an elective heart procedure, as many as 160,000 of which are probably inappropriate. Forty-five percent of those who have pump support during surgery develop what is known as "pump head," vernacular for diminished cognitive functions.

Commenting on the rush to operate, an editorial in the *New England Journal of Medicine* put part of the blame for these unnecessary procedures on heart disease patients, who often insist on the intervention (66). On the other hand, when someone's confronted with the warning, "You're going to die without this operation," the choice does seem rather moot.

It is important to recognize, too, that every scoundrel needs a foil. Without customers, medical exploiters would be out of business. But the supply of eager supplicants at the doors of the shadow practitioners seems endless. As mentioned earlier, one of my prime areas of interest is aging, which has had its generous quota of pseudo-practitioners promising salvation in a pill bottle or in an elixir of sheep or monkey glands. The immortality hucksters have scarcely missed a beat and prey energetically on the supplicants. An entire issue of the *Journal of Gerontology* was devoted to debunking their bogus mantra of eternal life (67).

Trust is a necessity for Medicine to assume its rightful place as a societal safeguard. Corruption cannot be tolerated.


## Symptom 5: Inefficiency

Physicists define efficiency as work divided by input. We adapt this to medicine to define efficiency as patient satisfaction divided by cost and other resources invested (such as time). Peak efficiency connotes the ideal functional state of a system, one that requires a minimum of time and energy and cost for the most work done—the most economical performance. When held to such a standard, Current Medicine of today reveals itself to be highly inefficient.

In its summary report, "National Scorecard of U.S. Health System Performance, 2008" (posted on July 17, 2008) (68), the Commonwealth Foundation found that "the U.S. health system continues to fall far short of what should be attainable, especially given the resources invested. Across 37 core indicators of performance, the U.S. achieves an overall score of 65 out of a possible 100 when comparing national averages with U.S. and international performance benchmarks. In the past two years it fell from 67 to 65." Further, "the quality of care is highly variable and opportunities are routinely missed to prevent disease, disability, hospitalization and mortality." Even more troubling, "the U.S. health system is on the wrong track. It fails to keep pace with gains in health outcomes achieved by leading countries. The U.S. ranks last out of 19 countries in a measure of mortality, amenable to medical response. Up to 101,000 fewer people would die prematurely if the leading benchmarks were obtained."

The United States was also the worst of seven countries surveyed in terms of difficulty getting to an emergency department. Inappropriate, wasteful, and fragmented care was repeatedly noted, as were excess administrative costs, which are three times higher than in other countries. Taken together, the surveys cited in the report are a stern indictment of the way we are performing as a medical system in terms of efficiency.

For all the gloss and PR offered up by the providers of Current Medicine, it is disheartening to learn that the hype is mostly just that. Most of us grew up in a world where American leadership was taken for granted, and that was clearly the case in medicine as well. American medicine is, however, no longer number one today, certainly not in terms of the objective measures of health care delivery. By the best of measures, it is not even number 2 or 3 or 4 or 5 or 6. It is not until we get to number 38 that the WHO international rating system finds the United States, snuggled between Costa Rica and Slovenia, ranked in total system merit. To be sure, sometimes our system hits a grand slam with high theater attending it. But the overall batting average is poor, putting us in the minor leagues of effectiveness.

There are a number of other measurements that an actuary can employ to estimate the efficiency and effectiveness of a nation's medical system. Longevity is the most obvious. On this score alone, the United States ranks 45th, below Bosnia and Herzegovina and Jordan, as well as most of Western Europe. Our life expectancy is 78.1, compared to Andorra's leading 83.5. Cuba ranks 56th, less than 1 year shorter than ours, and with 1% of the cost. Virtually all of the lowest-ranking countries are in sub-Saharan Africa, where AIDS plays a savage role. Overall, most countries are improving, but are improving faster than we are, so that we are still falling farther behind.

A footnote here is that we also lag in height statistics. Prof. John Komlos of the University of Munich has been studying population height in different eras (69). Two hundred years ago, the average Dutch male was 3 inches shorter than the average American. Now he is 3 inches taller, at 6-foot-1. At the time of the American Revolution, our soldiers were 2 inches taller than the British, 5-foot-9 versus 5-foot-7. Now the British men are half an inch taller, at 5-foot-10, than American men. According to Komlos, "America has gone from being the tallest nation in the world to the fattest."

Prof. George Maat of Leiden University is another height-ologist. He believes that stature represents "health, nutrition, living conditions, genetics" and is the easiest parameter to use to illuminate the conditions people are living in, "the best single indication of a nation's success" (70). So the United States lags behind in two related measurements, and it may be getting worse with regard to longevity. Several years ago, the CDC sent out a storm warning, forecasting that unless certain unhealthy trends in our country were reversed, we faced the first decline in national life expectancy since the founding of the republic.

A paper in *PLoS Medicine* in April 2008, "Reversal of Fortunes," indicates that this is already happening (71). Using statistics for life expectancy between 1961 and 1991, supplied by the Census Bureau and the Center for Health Statistics, the authors reported that in certain American counties, there was a 1.3-year decrease in life expectancy. This was the result of increased mortality from lung cancer, emphysema, diabetes, and a range of other noncommunicable diseases that were not compensated for by a decrease in cardiovascular mortality. Higher AIDS and homicide rates also contributed to the male decline.

But beyond longevity, the WHO report included assessments such as low-birthweight babies, disabilities, and of course cost. The organization's assessment of the American health care system is an embarrassment.

One of the effects of our medical system's inefficiency is the wide variation in care from place to place. Dartmouth's John Wennberg has set the standard in this area with his elegant studies showing the inconsistent pattern of medical care in the United States. In 1967, with a $350,000 grant from Lyndon Johnson, he began analyzing Medicare data to see how well hospitals and doctors were performing (72). "Our results were fascinating, because they ran completely counter to what conventional wisdom had said they would be," he wrote in *Health Affairs* in 2004 (73). "Everyone expected that we would clearly see under-care in rural hospital service areas remote from academic medical centers. But when we looked at the data, we found tremendous variation in every aspect of health care delivery, even among communities served by academic medical centers. We found the same thing when we compare health care in the Boston and New Haven communities served by some of the finest academic medical centers in the world. The basic premise that medicine is driven by science and by physicians, capable of making clinical decisions based on well-established fact and theory, was simply incompatible with the data we saw" (74).

In 1997 *Health Affairs* named Wennberg the most important health policy-maker in the past 25 years (75). Don Berwick called his work "the most important health services research of this century." Berwick and Wennberg are widely cited as claiming that fully one third of all medical expenses are wasted.

Wennberg recently retired as head of Dartmouth Medical School's Center for the Evaluative Clinical Sciences, which he had led since 1988. His work has been a foundation of the important *Dartmouth Atlas of Health Care*, an invaluable source of nationwide data (76). He has exploited Medicare data for his research, which involves mostly older people who use the system more and die more often. In fact, some of Wennberg's studies involve the cost of dying, which again shows marked regional differences, particularly in New York. Try not to die in New York: it is too expensive. Wennberg has devoted his career to showing how different New Haven is from Boston, how different Shreveport is from Portland. Even within a community, hospitals and office practices can differ by orders of magnitude.

For example, Medicare expenditures for the last 2 years of life of older patients average $40,000 in New Jersey and $23,700 in Idaho. New Jersey patients average 42 doctor visits in the last 6 months of life, compared with 17 in Utah. Patients in Hawaii spend 16.4 days of their last 6 months of life in the hospital, whereas Utah patients spend just 7.3 days. New Haven and Newark differ 100% in rates of prostate surgery. There is a 400% difference between the number of back surgeries in Manhattan and in Fort Myers. Rapid City and rural Ohio differ 34 times in the rate of breast reconstructive surgery after mastectomy.

A July 2008 posting by *Consumer Reports*, "Too Much Treatment," cites Wennberg's *Dartmouth Atlas* study of 4,732,448 Medicare patients in thousands of U.S. hospitals for the years 2001 to 2005. The patients suffered from serious illnesses, such as heart failure and cancer, in the last 2 years of their lives. In some parts of the country, patients got aggressive medical care, involving specialists and ordering of more tests and treatments. The costs of this treatment were two to three times greater than in areas with more conservative management schemes, but resulted in no longer survival or better quality of life. The aggressively treated group had more infections and generated more medical errors. Finally, the patients in the aggressive group reported less satisfaction with their care than those in the conservative one. *Consumer Reports* concludes that although some people equate more care with better care, in fact too much care may shorten your life.

In October 2004, Wennberg and his associates surveyed 77 of the 100 hospitals that *US News and World Report* included in their "best hospitals in

America" list and found evidence that more is not necessarily better, and in many cases is worse. Many blue-ribbon hospitals do not deserve their renown. One of my personal pieces of advice is, "If you want to get the inside dope on anyone or any organization, ask a nurse. They don't get their information from the headlines, and they know who really is best."

Posted on the Web site of Physicians for a National Health Program is an abstract of a *Health Affairs* article entitled "Evaluating the Efficiency of California Providers in Caring for Patients with Chronic Illness" (77). It reports the results of studies of hospitals in five regions of California from 1998 to 2003. In the last years of patients' lives, the hospitals in the Los Angeles area received 60% more reimbursement from Medicare for the same diagnosis than those in Sacramento. Actually, in some cases, Medicare paid four times as much in one region than in another for similar cases. Yet the report showed that there was no correlation between the quality and quantity of care and either costs or the level of patient satisfaction. The authors concluded that Medicare would have saved $1.7 billion if L.A.'s expenses had matched Sacramento's.

In the *Dartmouth Atlas*, Wennberg notes that "when the contents of the medical 'black box' are examined more closely, the type of medical service provided is often found to be strongly influenced by subjective factors related to the attitudes of the individual physician as much as by science." The Rand Corporation has reported that one in seven deaths attributable to heart disease, stroke, and pneumonia is preventable (78). The Office of Technology Assessment estimates that less than 20% of treatments have actually been shown to be effective.

## Symptom 6: Irrelevance

Any patient who enters the office with the number of complaints that our medical system exhibits qualifies for the diagnosis of total body pain. Total body pain, however, does not conform to any standard diagnostic category. It is not listed in any textbook. But to the experienced practitioner, someone with problems in every part of his or her body has a condition that does not lend itself to reductionist, or piecemeal, analysis, something we will talk more about later. By definition, total body pain is a systemic problem. And because it requires a systemic analysis, we must stand back and look outside the jumbled box of Current Medicine.

As we ponder Current Medicine's list of symptoms—cost, inequity, harmfulness, corruption, and inefficiency—it is not until we arrive at irrelevance that we encounter a problem that is not fundamentally administrative in nature. The first five symptoms are theoretically susceptible to technical remedies, but the symptom of irrelevance makes us wonder whether there is something more profound going on, something that cannot be fixed by administrative action. The first five symptoms might seem to be fixable by some belt tightening or loosening, by basically minor quantitative adjustments. But as we review the several powerful examples of irrelevance, we see the reality: Current Medicine is failing. Despite a huge treasury, peerless technology, and the leading scientific enterprise in the world, our life expectancy and system performance standards are regularly judged to be inferior. I use the term "irrelevance" to signify a complete disconnect between Americans' health and our health care system. There is, fundamentally, no relation between the two.

Noted medical economist Robert Evans recounts the situation a few years ago when nurses in Los Angeles went on strike for higher wages (79). At the same time, the state health commission ruled that there were too many empty beds in Los Angeles hospitals. The city had more beds than it needed. "Isn't it strange that we are unable to afford something that we don't need in the first place?" Evans observed. This cogent remark applies perfectly to the American medical mess. The tools and personnel we possess, as elegant as they may be, are irrelevant to the ultimate task of assuring human potential.

The chief SOS signals on medicine's unhealthy horizon come from aging and "diabesity," a term coined by former surgeon general C. Everett Koop (80). These are new problems that had no constituency until recently. Now these twin epidemics occupy a major portion of the medical horizon. They cause millions of deaths and untold misery, and they cost trillions of dollars. The relief agency at hand, Current Medicine, is powerless to address them. Its paradigm is wrong.

Current Medicine lacks the philosophical, moral, and scientific conceptual framework that would make it capable of helping. It is called upon to make a house call for symptoms attributable to aging and diabetes. It reaches into its black bag for a remedy. In the bag are the fundamental tools of the medical-industrial complex, surgery and pills. These two treatments represent nearly all of Current Medicine's $2.5 trillion annual budget, but they are powerless against aging and diabetes. This is not to say that Current Medicine does not prescribe surgery and pills for these two conditions—it does, extravagantly. But the conceptual framework, the theoretical platform, the science, does not match the new necessity that aging and diabetes create. Instead of the current model, diabetes and aging require a treatment in which prevention supersedes cure. But this approach is not in Current Medicine's black bag.

So there we have our case—a terribly flawed medical system exhibiting multiple serious symptoms. A diagnostician hardly knows where or how to begin the workup. One of the most valuable ways of getting insight into the troubled patient is to take a careful history.

Whenever I sought to diagnose a patient, I always felt that getting that person's medical history was the most important part of the exam. Futurists, of course, predict that this will soon be obsolete: All the patient will have to do is to pass through a high-tech-wizardry portal and we will know what is wrong; no talking or touching will be required. I doubt that any of this is near at hand. So in searching for the diagnosis of Current Medicine, I think a review of Medicine's history is in order (1).

Who was the first doctor, and what was her job? What were her office hours?

Or did doctors perhaps exist before humans came into being? In her lovely book *The Sacred Depths of Nature*, Ursula Goodenough tells the story of a young bonobo chimp who injures a bird while playing with it (2): "She picked up the comatose body, carried it with her to the top of a tree and opened out her hand. When the bird still lay there limply she wrapped her legs around the tree trunk, held the bird by its wings, and then opened and closed the wings several times, apparently trying to help it start to fly." Such a primal expression of caring seems deeply rooted in our nature.

The French philosopher Henri Bergson said that man is alone in realizing that he is subject to illness. Animals cruise through their lives oblivious to the slings and arrows of fortune. They do not know when they need a doctor.

Nonetheless, animals have evolved prodigious survival skills. Nature heals most things on her own (3).

## Health and Our Earliest Ancestors

When and how did humankind develop a healing tradition? Just when did the idea of medical care arise? Our Paleolithic grandparents shared with the other wild animals certain common causes of death: starvation, violence (predation, accidents, murder, war), and infection. The last, however, was not as serious, because the hunter-gatherer era was characterized by sparse population density (one person per 10 square kilometers) and bacteria's reliance on population crowding to maximize their potency. Wild animals and our hunter-gatherer ancestors were prone to infections by protozoan parasites, but such infection was chronic and not thought to contribute to group mortality. The bacteria and viruses that would come to dominate human disease patterns for 10,000 years were still in the future.

Predation was clearly a constant threat. Tennyson's "nature red in tooth and claw" accompanied each dawn and every sunset. Lucy, our earliest ancestor, and her relatives were small, slow, and unarmed with any lethal bodily equipment, so they were obviously at a disadvantage when faced with the major predators loose on the Serengeti.

After guesstimating the number of deaths due to murder, war, and sacrifice against the cumulative world population to date of 151 billion (the area under the curve in Fig. 3.1), it's clear that most of our number have succumbed to less violent endings (4). Thus, food availability emerges as the principal threat to health for our earliest ancestors. A look at the world population figures reveals the power of Malthusian law. In 1798, a British minister named Thomas Malthus proclaimed that humans' reproductive capacity increases exponentially, while food capacity proceeds arithmetically (5). The small world population at the time of the Agricultural Revolution clearly illustrates this fact.

If even a small fraction of our ancestors had had stomachs that were full enough to consider reproducing, we would by now be up to our eyebrows in people. Jared Diamond projected that if a colony of 100 people grew at a rate of 1.1% per year, its population would reach 10 million within a thousand years (6). And since Lucy, we have 5 million years to account for.

An important but unrecognized biological law applies here: the Principle of the Least (7). Briefly stated, it maintains that when we retrace the evolutionary history of any species, it is not sufficient to presume an environmental setting similar to the present. It is necessary to apply the worst environmental conditions,

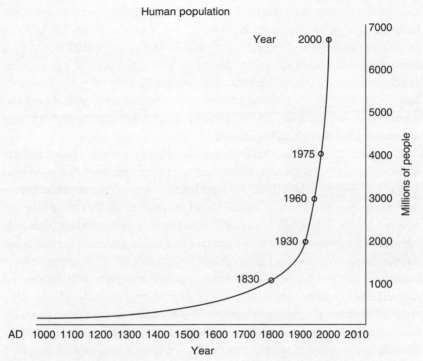

**Figure 3.1** World population.

because for our genetic line to have survived until the present (99.9% of all prior species are now extinct), our ancestors' genes had to squeeze through some tight fits.

The tightest evolutionary test for our ancestors was those single years in 100 or 1,000 or 10,000 when the Serengeti was parched and scorched and they were hungry. Our survival depended on our ancestors' ability to catch and eat that remaining wildebeest down in the Olduvai Gorge.

I love to recreate this picture for crowds of runners in Boston or New York or wherever on the eve of a marathon run. "The sounds of the footsteps we'll be hearing will not simply be our own," I tell them, "but the echoes of those of millions of others whose survival depended entirely on their ability to run."

Food and the ability to move are synonymous. In paleo-times, when older people were no longer able to move, they were abandoned, not through cruelty, but by the demands of necessity. Yet we survived, not only through the Serengeti famines, but through thousands of others (8).

Accidents were also common. Many Paleolithic bones testify to the extreme mechanical stresses they endured. Someone likened the skeletal remains of a Neanderthal to those of a rodeo rider in terms of the punishment and breakage they suffered. Stanford's Richard Klein is a recognized authority on the Neanderthals. In his textbook *The Human Career* (9) he notes: "The skeletal pathologies and injuries that show that Neanderthals lived risky lives and aged early also reveal a strikingly human feature of their social life. The La Chapelle-aux-Saints and Shanidar I individuals, for example, must have been severely incapacitated and would have died even earlier without substantial help and care from their comrades." So we can infer that Neanderthals cared for their disadvantaged fellows 50,000 years ago.

One less-than-evident threat to our ancestors' survival was childbirth. In her chapter "Evolutionary Obstetrics" in *Evolutionary Medicine*, Wenda Trevathan describes the skeletal changes that accompanied our descent from the trees to the open savanna. Unlike our other primate cousins, who have lots of room for the offspring's head to emerge, the large human head is severely compromised in the mother's birth canal (10); this is known as craniopelvic disproportion. Further, the human infant must rotate en route so that it faces away from the mother, which potentially compromises the first breath and requires assistance from another party at the moment of birth. Unlike other animals, humans give birth preferably with an attendant present, which, as statistics show, increases the chances of survival. Taking all this into consideration, it is reasonable to suggest that the first real physician, the first person to assert and assure human potential, was a midwife, an early obstetrician.

But the first definitive evidence of real "medical" treatment dates to 10,000 years ago. Skulls from that period show the indisputable marks of trephining, or boring holes in the skull with flint as a way of treating headaches or insanity, or preventing blindness, or letting out demons. Human sacrifice came to be a standard offering to appease the unhappy agents of disease.

The earliest known written medical record was an Egyptian obelisk from 2400 BC, well after the Agricultural Revolution had begun (11). The Agricultural Revolution itself produced important transitions: it signaled the historic moment when our ancestors no longer had to chase their food or be chased as food, but instead stayed at home in a group. Farming became the principal occupation, and due to a steady supply of adequate calories, a population explosion began. With it came crowding and "crowd diseases," the inevitable surge in infections that came to dominate the next 17,000 years of medical history. The occurrence of virulence has continued to ravage humankind periodically: consider that over 95% of the population in northwest China died of plague in the year 310.

Thomas McKeown projects that until 300 years ago, two to three of every 10 children died before their first birthday, five to six by age 6, and seven before maturity (3). Death was a constant companion, usually abrupt, often violent, and always unexplained. Astrologers and mystics blamed epidemics on cosmic events; demons and witches pre-empted rationality. Medicine's mission of asserting and assuring our potential was governed by superstition and ignorance.

It is generally conceded that primitive man regarded sickness as a supernatural phenomenon (12). He believed that any afflictions were due to the maleficent influence of gods, the black magic of wizards, the evil eye of an enemy, the offended spirits of dead men or animals or even plants. Animism came to be the basis of medical folklore. Early preventive medicine was a practice of fetishes and spells, a propitiating or cajoling of gods and spirits, white magic pitted against black, a hocus-pocus of the supernatural. Illness was regarded as punishment for sin, "a whip in the hand of God." Man's efforts to prevent it were an attempt to restrain the devil; to tease, bribe, or coerce the spirits to stay their hands.

In his renowned book *Persuasion and Healing*, noted Johns Hopkins psychiatrist Jerome Frank (13) writes about the role of shamans in confronting human ignorance about disease and health. What shamans offer is a curious mix of pantomime, prestidigitation, and empirical knowledge in societies where illnesses are viewed as "symbolic expressions of internal conflicts or of disturbed relationships to others, or both. They may be attributed to soul loss, possession by an evil spirit, the magical insertion of a harmful body by a sorcerer, or the machinations of offended malicious ghosts…. Although many societies recognize that certain illnesses may have a natural cause, this does not exclude the simultaneous role of supernatural ones. A broken leg may be recognized as caused by a fall from a tree, but the cause of the fall may have been an evil thought or a witch's curse." Shamans, interestingly, tend to reject people whom they feel they cannot cure. Voodoo death practices endure until today (14).

## Babylon and Egypt

As civilization advanced, observant individuals began to intuit that filth and contamination were common precursors to illness. "Cleanliness is next to godliness" is an ancient truism (15). The earliest known plumbing was in Babylon; excavations unearthed a pyramid in which 1,300 feet of copper drainpipe had been installed 2,500 years before the birth of Christ. Other sanitation relics give evidence of sensitivity to public health (16). In the Bible, Moses is preoccupied with sanitation. The practice of kosher meat preparation was instrumental in avoiding tuberculosis.

Hammurabi (1728–1686 BC), the sixth king of the first Babylonian dynasty, presided over some of the earliest recorded medical practices. Scraps of records describe Babylonian medicine in 2000 BC. Sore eyes, for instance, were (and still are) common in the lands of the *khamsin*, the hot dry wind that blows out of the Arabian desert. The eye trouble was ascribed to the demon of the south-west wind, who was represented as an eagle with the head of a dog and the claws of a lion. The demon was supposedly frightened by the ugliness of his own image, so people would set carvings of him outside their homes to ward off the afflictions he brought. To treat sore eyes, the priest/doctor would prescribe a drink of a cut-up onion mixed with beer. This was obviously to encourage tears, which we now know have germicidal properties. Then the eyes were to be assuaged with oil (17). Several papyri from nearby Egypt represent the oldest surviving medical books. The Elders Papyrus, ca. 1550 BC, is more than 20 meters long and describes dozens of diseases and hundreds of healing compounds. The Egyptian physician specialized in a single part of the body, the vanguard, it seems, of our era of the medical specialist. Out of this milieu arose Imhotep.

Imhotep was famed as a priest/doctor. In *Evolution of Modern Medicine*, Sir William Osler described him as "the first figure of a physician to stand out clearly from the mists of antiquity" (18). Imhotep diagnosed and treated more than 200 diseases, including 15 diseases of the abdomen, 11 of the bladder, 29 of the eyes, and 18 of the skin, hair, nails and tongue. He treated tuberculosis, gallstones, appendicitis, gout, and arthritis, and he also performed surgery and practiced some dentistry. He extracted medicine from plants, and he also knew the position and function of the vital organs.

The Egyptians placed a great deal of faith in drugs, using the poppy and the hyoscyamus, a common botanical that drug firms use as a source of alkaloids, among other active ingredients. Arthritis, tuberculosis, and worms are evident in their antiquities. Egyptian medicine was the first glimpse of the science of medicine, which would wait another 2,000 years to reach full flower, until the Greek enlightenment and Hippocrates.

## The Greeks and the Romans

The single greatest moment of enlightenment in medical science arrived in Greece in the period 700–300 BC, the Golden Age of Pericles. Out of the murky mist of ignorance, groping efforts to explain the unexplained were born. The Greek mind provided a beacon in the darkness. In his book *The Passion of the Western Mind,* Richard Tarnas observed that "the Greeks were the first to see the world as something to be known" (19). The Greek mind was "curious, innovative, critical, intensely engaged with the main events of life and death, searching for order and meaning, yet skeptical of conventional verities." The Greeks' brilliance gave birth to both democracy and science. It is no coincidence that these two fundamental pillars of human civilization emerged at the same time and in the same place.

This was also the era of the Oracle of Delphi, another proof of the Greeks' original and epic approach to all things human. Her influence eventually declined, but two of her precious teachings remain. First, "Hold this principle most holy: Know thyself." This commandment, incidentally, is central to my definition of medicine's mission of asserting human potential, which is clearly possible only if we possess self-knowledge. The second precept was "everything in moderation." This principle effectively describes the Golden Mean, a tenet that is basic to much of Aristotelian philosophy and is visibly demonstrated in the construction of the Parthenon.

Equally important were the Greek philosophers. Historian Richard Tarnas called Plato's thought "the single most important foundation for the evolution of the Western mind." Plato equipped all subsequent generations with his inspired vision of man as an autonomous being who becomes what he does. Aristotle emphasized the power of man's reason to comprehend the cosmos. And to assist that power, he introduced empirical experimentation as a means of adding to the storehouse of knowledge, becoming one of the first to perform dissections of macaque monkeys (human autopsies or dissections were forbidden). Earlier, knowledge of the human body, both its anatomy and its function, had been extremely crude. Establishing known parameters for health and illness was a critical step in the subsequent development of medicine.

Hippocrates adopted the Aristotelian approach of direct inquiry. Enlightened self-interest, or knowing oneself, became the dominant canon. Hippocrates and Aristotle insisted on the assiduous pursuit of the first principles, which lay hidden beneath the clutter of everyday human endeavor. Hippocrates enshrined his doctrines in The Corpus, a collection of 60 works on various topics that is the source of great scholarly debate. The central thesis is that knowledge is obtained through reasoned thought, and not through revelation. The Hippocratic Oath, which is given in numerous medical school graduation ceremonies, stresses physician selflessness and the primacy of nature's ways.

Illustrative of the Greek approach to medicine is the legend of Asclepius (20). Legend has it he was Apollo's son, born of a mortal mother. His mother took on a lover while she was pregnant with him, which was not a smart idea, because when it came to light, the gods punished her by setting her on fire soon after she gave birth. Apollo then placed the motherless infant in the care of a centaur named Chiron. Chiron was known throughout Greece as a great teacher, and as he raised Asclepius, he taught him about health and disease.

When Asclepius came of age, the gods charged him with caring for the health of all Greek mortals. He fathered many children, several of whom helped with the family business, including two daughters. The older, Hygeia, washed and scrubbed her father's patients, which helped protect the mortals' health, so much so that she came to represent health itself, giving rise to the word *hygiene*. Hygeia came to represent the virtue of a sane life in a pleasant environment, the ideal of *mens sano in corpore sano*—a clean mind in a sound body. And in concert with this was the notion that the body tends to heal itself, *Vis medicatrix naturae*. Nature heals. (People whose diseases are prevented as opposed to cured may never really appreciate what has been done for them. The gods may have been pleased with Asclepius's pursuit of hygiene to maintain health, but, as might be said to be true today, mortals would barely have been aware of his hygienist powers.)

Asclepius's other daughter, Panacea, represented the power to cure those who were already sick. Hygeia and Panacea thus represent an age-old dichotomy: prevention versus cure. The ancient Greeks understood better than we do today that these are both ways of treating disease. Panacea built her reputation as the great healer. She mastered the use of the knife and studied the curative values of plants. Eventually, her disciples outpaced those of Hygeia. Outside her temples, mortals waited in long lines to be cured. She changed the way the mortals thought about their health. Health did not occur naturally or as a result of cleanliness: it was a gift they obtained at the hands of a physician. René DuBos, formerly a scientist at Rockefeller Institute and a philosopher-humanist, commented that to ward off disease and recover health, man as a rule finds it easier to depend on the healer than to attempt the more difficult task of living wisely (21).

Any history of health medicine must also take into account the ancient Greeks' embrace of athletics. The Olympic Games were said to have been founded by Hercules, a son of Zeus (22). The first authenticated year was 776 BC. The ancient games were held every 4 years for 1,200 years until the Roman emperor discontinued them in 393 AD, only to be reignited some 1,500 years later. Homer described the many events of the games, including boxing. The games were extremely popular and came to represent the epitome of health and superior performance.

In contrast to the Greeks, physicians in Roman days were usually freed slaves, foreigners, and persons of low social standing (23). It was Galen the Roman who perpetuated the Hippocratic medical ideal. He adopted many of the Greek precepts and wrote extensively enough that the Greek Hippocratic school remained virtually intact for 2,000 years.

## The Middle Ages and Beyond

In the 13th century, Roger Bacon (1210–1273) took up the torch and spoke boldly against unreason, carrying Aristotle's fundamental outlook to the age (24). But during the Dark Ages and the Middle Ages and beyond, religious zealotry subverted the liberation of the questioning mind. Ignatius of Loyola preached that man should sacrifice the intellect to God. The Church resented, restricted, and subjugated inquiry into man's nature. In this, the devil was a convenient ally. The study of anatomy became a sin: everything was a sin, because sin was the sales product of the Church.

During this long, dark period, humankind was buffeted by the new scourges of bacterial and viral epidemics and the cultural deprivation of a cruel feudal system, one substantial byproduct of which was insufficient food for the populace, which suffered from famines of major proportions. Even more significant was chronic malnourishment, which led to reduced resistance to infections. Vitamin deficiency diseases—notably beriberi, scurvy, and pellagra—added to the miseries. Just look at those suits of armor in the world's museums. They are tiny, proof positive of how underfed the people of the time were.

But the Church maintained that it alone could ease the world's miseries. The Bible, after all, said so. Read Deuteronomy: "It shall come to pass ... If thou will not listen to the voice of the Lord thy God ... the Lord shall make the pestilence cleave unto thee, until it has consumed thee from off the land, whither thou goest to possess it. The Lord shall smite thee with a consumption, and with a fever, and with an inflammation, and with an extreme burning, and with the sword, and with blasting, and with mildew ... and they shall pursue thee until thou perish."

Thus leprosy became a purgatory on earth, curable only by the Lord. Gruesome descriptions of its horrible ravages terrorized the penitents. Death was the Church's trump card, because its finality kept all in constant fear. Anyone who dared question the Church was threatened with eternal hellfire and reminded that only the Church held the keys to heaven (25).

It is fortunate for us that this extraordinary scheme left behind some of history's greatest art as a byproduct of the power of the Church. But this was not always in full communion with the Church's exclusive claim to modulate sin. Dr. F. L. Meshberger published an article in 1990 in *JAMA* entitled "An Interpretation of Michelangelo's Creation of Adam Based on Neuroanatomy" (26). Dr. Meshberger discovered an extraordinary feature of the God figure in the central panel of creation, where God's forefinger touches Adam's. He presents indisputable evidence that the specific contour lines of the God figure correspond precisely with the anatomic features of the sagittal section of the human brain in fine detail. The inevitable conclusion is that Michelangelo made this blasphemous political statement that God is actually a representation of the human brain rather than the reverse. My minor reading of Michelangelo's life indicates that he was having huge struggles with the Pope's authority at the time of his painting. This caricature was his forceful statement of rebellion. We are informed that Michelangelo performed much covert examination of corpses to inform his glorious art. Never has the incredible beauty of the human body been more magnificently expressed.

Meanwhile, people went hungry. And then came the violent eruption of plague, the Black Death. The great pestilence of 1347 to 1357, possibly of Chinese origin, killed 20 million people in Europe, a quarter of the entire population. Florence's population fell from 100,000 to 38,000. Boccaccio (1313–1375) described the effects of the plague in *The Decameron*, a collection of tales told by refugees from Florence (27). Such was the cruelty of heaven, and to a great degree of man, that between March 1348 and the following July, more than 100,000 human beings lost their lives within the walls of Florence alone because of the plague's ravages and the barbarous behavior of the survivors toward the sick. It was generally believed that God had unleashed the plague to punish humankind for its sins. Physicians sought to protect themselves by donning long gowns and masks stuffed with aromatic herbs to protect them from inhaling vicious vapors.

The Dark Ages represented the nadir of medical competence. Consider the case of King Charles II of England. At 8 o'clock in the morning of February 2, 1685, while being shaved in his bedroom, he fell backward with a sudden cry and suffered a violent convulsion. He became unconscious, then over the next few days rallied once or twice, but finally died. Dr. Scarburgh, one of 14 physicians called to treat the stricken king, recorded the efforts to cure the patient (28):

> As the first step in treatment, the king was bled to the extent
> of a pint from a vein in his right arm. Next the shoulder was
> incised, and the area cupped to suck out an additional
> 8 ounces of blood. After this the drugging began. An emetic
> and purgative were administered and soon after a second
> purgative. This was followed by an enema containing
> antimony, sacred bitters, rock salt, mallow leaves, beet root,
> chamomile flowers, fennel seed, linseed, cinnamon,
> cardamom seed, saffron, cochineal and aloes. The enema
> was repeated in two hours and a purgative given. The King's
> head was shaved and a blister was raised on the scalp.
> A sneezing powder of hellebore root was administered, and

also a powder of cowslip flowers to "strengthen his brain...."
For external treatment, a plaster of Burgundy pitch and
pigeon dung was applied to the king's feet. The bleeding and
purging continued and the following medicaments were
added: melon seeds, slippery elm, black cherry water and
extract of flowers of lime, lily of the valley, peony, lavender,
and dissolved pearls. Still to come were gentian roots,
nutmeg, quinine, and cloves.

The King's condition did not improve. In fact, it grew worse,
and in the emergency 40 drops of extract of human skull
were administered to allay convulsions .... Then, after an
ill-fated night his serene majesty's strength seemed exhausted
to such a degree that the whole assembly of physicians lost
all hope, and became despondent. Still, so as not to appear
to fail in doing their duty in any detail, they brought into
play the most active cordial. As a sort of grand summary to
this pharmaceutical debauch, a mixture of Raleigh's
antidote, pearl julep, and ammonia was forced down the
throat of the dying king.

Some have said that Charles's death at the hands of his doctors was far
crueler than his father's death at the hands of the executioner. It took centuries
for Medicine to work itself out of this miserable state of passivity and ignorance.

Gradually, with the Renaissance and the Enlightenment, the veil started to
lift. Time slowly helped loosen the absolute proscription against mutilating the
human body lest it prevent reincarnation. The pursuit of anatomical dissection,
or *autopsy* ("see yourself"), secretly pursued by Leonardo da Vinci, Michelangelo,
and Albrecht Dürer, vastly expanded knowledge of the body's workings.
Leonardo did 750 anatomical drawings, "Passing the night hours in the company of these corpses quartered and flayed and horrible to behold" (29).
Ultimately, the Enlightenment produced the great scientists Isaac Newton,
Francis Bacon (Roger's son), and William Harvey, who was the first to describe
the workings of the circulatory system.

Around the same time that anatomic competence was added to the medical
lexicon, surgery was developed by Ambroise Paré (1510–1590) in Paris (30).
He derived his skill from service in the army, which provided all manner of
reconstructive opportunities. The surgeon's main task beyond lancing and
suturing became bloodletting, which was a leftover from the Hippocratic
tradition of unbalanced humors.

But for the most part, up to that point, the medical profession as a whole, such as it was, mostly watched and waited. Through the twists and turns of recorded history, medicine was essentially a passive observer, not an active participant, developing little in the way of new cures.

Hospitals as we know them grew out of Christian charity. During the great Crusade, from 1096 to 1291, numerous hospitals for the sick sprang up like motel chains along the way to the Holy Land. This was not necessarily a boon to the sick. Hospitals such as the original Hôtel Dieu in Paris, founded in 651 by the Bishop of Paris and acknowledged as the oldest hospital still in existence, contained 2,000 beds. In 1788, the death rate in hospitals was 25%, and sometimes eight patients occupied a single bed. The hospital movement advanced at a great pace, although at any given moment it was difficult to assess whether this was a benefit or a threat. Often the trip to the hospital was one-way.

Curative efforts remained stuck with a smattering of botanicals of uncertain good and unpracticed effects. Danger was a constant companion. With regard to the drugs, Oliver Wendell Holmes wrote, "Without opium which the Creator Himself seems to prescribe for we often see the scarlet poppy growing in the cornfields as if it were foreseen that wherever there is hunger to be fed, there must also be pain to be soothed. Throw out a few specifics, throw out wine, which our art did not discover and which is a food, and the vapors which produce the miracle of anesthesia and I firmly believe that if the whole Materia Medica as now used could be sunk to the bottom of the sea it would be all the better for mankind, and all the worse for the fishes" (31).

By the 1800s, the average physician had learned most of what he knew on the job, with possibly a stint of apprenticeship along the way. He cobbled therapies together from folk remedies, alcohol-based tonics, sexual enhancers, hair promoters, age delayers, and wart removers. There were no regulations, and no certification. Inasmuch as there was no true science within Medicine, what succeeded was an art, aided immeasurably by the placebo effect. Most illnesses are self-limiting, so physicians often played for time and hoped to get credit for any positive results that may or may not have been due to their ministrations (32,33).

## New World Medicine

On the other side of the Atlantic, a new nation was being born. Its birth was another triumph of revolt against authoritarian strictures. The New World was to provide Medicine the stage on which it might stand with pride as an active participant in humankind's larger destiny.

At the same time, however, the free-wheeling entrepreneurial American character made early New World Medicine a shadowy affair. Quacks and ridiculous nostrums prevailed. A trip to the doctor was a hazardous undertaking. There was only the faintest glimmer that Medicine might be a profession worthy of respect. Anyone who was so inclined could appropriate the title of doctor, and many did. Opportunism abounded. Physicians, surgeons, and apothecaries jostled for advantage and fees. The surgeon became distinct from the barber only in 1745. The apothecary actually provided the bulk of medical advice. Most physicians were part-time itinerants who eked out a living by inventive charades of little or no medical value.

Benjamin Franklin helped transform those charades into a systematic and professional field of study: he was an exemplar of the Greek spirit of reasoned inquiry. While certainly not a physician in any formal sense, Franklin contributed greatly to the advancement of the science and art of Medicine. He complained, presciently, "I love science so much that I regret that I was born too soon." His *Poor Richard's Almanac,* published in 1732, was filled with medical information and drawings (34). With French physician friends, he advocated for the removal of the shackles that had chained mental patients to the walls of Paris asylums for 300 years.

On the other hand, there was the other Benjamin, Benjamin Rush. He was a contemporary of Franklin's, one of three physicians who signed the Declaration of Independence. Rush was born in Philadelphia, but went to Edinburgh for medical training (35). There he absorbed the remaining tenets of Galenic/Hippocratic theory that disease had no specific origin in the body, but occurred as a result of a systemic disturbance caused by an imbalance in the four basic humors: blood, phlegm, and yellow and black bile. Rush taught more than 2,000 medical students and basically disavowed nature's power to cure. He openly urged closing all hospitals, which he saw as citadels of pestilence. Bleeding was his primary therapy; it consisted of opening a vein in the arm with a blade, and inducing catharsis by administering heavy doses of mercury chloride, a powerful laxative. Rush further advised that these therapies should be used with courage and until the patient was unconscious and began to salivate. He prescribed this regimen for all conditions, including colds and a runny nose due to allergies.

Rush had a hand in helping America's first black physician, James Derham. Derham, born in Philadelphia in 1757, was a slave who was indentured to three physicians, one of whom encouraged him to become a physician. Working as a medical assistant and apothecary, Derham saved enough money to buy his freedom, and in 1783 opened a medical practice in New Orleans. There he met

Rush, who persuaded him to move back to Philadelphia. Derham became an expert in throat diseases (36).

Early America had its own version of the physician-aided death of England's King Charles II. On December 12, 1799, George Washington returned from a recreational ride complaining of a sore throat, for which he sought medical attention (37). Over the next two days, he was bled four times, and given calomel (a laxative) and tartar (an emetic). When he did not improve, a young doctor suggested a revolutionary new treatment to help Washington's labored breathing—a tracheotomy, which most likely would have further hastened his death. Of course, the young doctor was overruled by his elders, who applied blistering agents to Washington's legs and feet instead. Washington died on December 14, killed more by medical practice than by any medical condition.

Two developments, however, helped the advancement of medical professionalism in the New World. The first was the recognition (again, the Greeks had pointed the way) that religion and medicine were two separate things. The second was the grudging respect granted to the first medical schools.

John Morgan (1735–1781) was an Edinburgh, Scotland, graduate who came to America and in 1765 started America's first medical school at the University of Pennsylvania. Harvard's was founded in 1782. Harvard Medical School provided two winters of lectures and a third year of apprenticeship, leading to the practice of medicine seven years later. Ten percent of the MDs of this era were also preachers. Of the 4,000 "doctors" in early America, only 400 had any medical training. Slowly, that would change.

By the time of the Civil War, American Medicine was still mired in an unholy enterprise of trial and error, mostly error (38). During that convulsive war, the Northern armies employed 11,000 physicians, mostly engaged in treating 500,000 cases of diarrhea per year and 1.4 million cases of malaria resulting in 15,000 deaths. Their additional chore was amputation, which was performed more than 30,000 times over the course of the conflict. Despite this total, more soldiers probably died from not having an amputation than from having one. Overall 600,000 men were killed in the Civil War, and another 600,000 wounded and disfigured. One million soldiers were taken to hospitals that were characterized as "the sinks of human life." They probably killed more than they saved.

The one positive development to come out of Civil War medicine was the introduction of ether anesthesia in 1846. This was a major medical advance that resulted largely from a series of fumbling serendipities. William Clark, an American doctor, was aware of an old German mixture (sweet oil of vitriol) with properties similar to nitrous oxide and used it for a successful dental extraction with ether in January 1842. Another Boston dentist, William Morton, had used ether on his pet dog, himself, and a patient to sound effect, so in October 1846, he persuaded John Warren at the Massachusetts General Hospital, previously disheartened by his experience with nitrous oxide, to use ether before the surgical removal of a neck tumor. This successful occasion is marked by a plaque at the MGH. Prior to general anesthesia, surgery had been a brutal undertaking combining sheer strength and speed to limit the patient's tortuous sufferings (39).

Ether, however, was extremely irritating and frequently caused nausea and vomiting, so it was soon displaced by chloroform. James Sampson, a professor of surgery at Edinburgh, had been experimenting with different anesthetic compounds when one of his students knocked over a bottle of chloroform, putting the entire class to sleep. Simpson thereafter employed it in his practice to good effect. Hearing this, John Snow, the man who had halted an epidemic of cholera in London by removing the handle of the Broad Street water pump, administered chloroform to Queen Victoria when she gave birth to Prince Leopold on August 7, 1853. She recalled the effect as "smoothing, quieting, and delightful beyond measure." Thus general inhaled anesthesia became a cornerstone of surgical practice. This was a major advance.

## Pasteur and the Birth of Modern Medicine

Pain, as awful as it was, was not the principal threat from surgery: that credential belonged to infection. The ancient Greeks were occasionally aware of the need for antisepsis, and through the centuries a number of chemicals were promoted for the care of wounds, but no real progress was made against infection until the mid-19th century. At that time, Vienna's Allgemeines Krankenhaus, or general hospital (where my father studied after graduating from Harvard Medical School in 1919), had two obstetrical services, one attended by medical students and the other by students in midwifery. The mortality in the midwifery ward was 3%; in the medical student ward, it was 30%. In 1847, Ignaz Semmelweis (1818–1865), an assistant physician, concluded that this was the result of the medical students coming directly from autopsies to the labor room. Semmelweis instructed physicians to wash their hands, and mortality rates immediately plummeted, although no one really understood why, as germs were still an unknown. Only a few years later, during the Crimean War in 1854, Florence Nightingale became a medical heroine as she almost single-handedly dealt with more than 2,000 wounded soldiers in closed-in, filthy wards using soap and a scrub brush and insisting on cleanliness. Thanks to her efforts, the death rate fell from 40% to 2%.

Then came Louis Pasteur (40). Born in 1822, the son of a peasant tanner, Pasteur earned his doctor of sciences degree in 1847 at the age of 25. His famous process of pasteurization arose from his efforts to prevent the kinds of illnesses caused by sour milk and bad wine that afflicted many in his day. Pasteur's chemical observation convinced him that the bad wine and milk were both caused by a living organism and did not occur spontaneously, as most organic chemists of the time maintained. He meticulously confirmed his theory through a series of experiments, and further demonstrated that heating destroyed the harmful bacteria. On February 18, 1878, Pasteur presented his germ theory of infection to the French Academy of Medicine. It spread quickly and was widely acclaimed.

Pasteur's other great contribution was the rabies vaccine, which he developed in experiments on rabbits and dogs. On July 6, 1885, 9-year-old Joseph Meister was brought to Pasteur's door. The boy had been bitten 15 times 2 days earlier by a dog thought to be rabid. Pasteur, haunted by the memory of the screams of victims of a wolf attack in his childhood village, didn't hesitate to initiate the painful series of 14 injections of increasing virulence. The boy did not develop any symptoms. Neither did a 14-year-old shepherd who had been severely bitten as he protected other children from a rabid dog. Over the next 15 months, more than 2,000 people were treated with Pasteur's vaccine, and more than 20,000 over the next decades. In 1950, a 10-year study revealed that only 0.6% of those treated with the vaccine treated died.

So Pasteur joins Aristotle and Hippocrates as a giant in the history of Medicine. The Greeks had asserted that health and illness were prompted by natural processes, but they lacked knowledge of the agency behind disease. Pasteur provided this with the germ theory. Modern medicine was born of this dual parenthood.

Elsewhere in Paris, another scientist, Claude Bernard (1813–1878) embarked upon securing his seat in the medical pantheon (41). Bernard taught us how the body works. His contention was that disease was caused by the body's faulty adaptation to the external environment, an insight the Greeks had had 2,000 years before. He was particularly struck by the constancy (*fixité*) of the workings of the *milieu interieure*, the interior environment, an insight that led the great American physiologist, Walter Cannon, to propose the term "homeostasis" for the body's capacity to balance itself when perturbed, which he described in his 1932 book, *The Wisdom of the Body* (42).

Bernard looked into how the different bodily systems functioned under highly controlled conditions. Experimenting on animals, he tied things off and watched what happened. He placed tubes in arteries and veins and measured the changes that resulted when different maneuvers were carried out. He clipped nerves and checked on saliva flow and temperature change.

From hundreds of experiments, Bernard concluded that the multiple inter-related functions of the body constituted an organized whole that exhibited a remarkable stability when the environment was severely manipulated. He maintained that sickness is often the result of the body trying to maintain itself and sustain life, continually attempting to restore the physiological condition when it is disturbed. Bernard's work eventually led to the field of endocrinol-ogy, showing how the body's many glands do and do not work. He insisted that physiology is the science of life and must be the scientific basis of medicine. In this, he added greatly to medicine's job description of asserting human potential. "I feel convinced," he prophesied, "that there will come a day when physiologists, poets, and philosophers will all speak the same language" (41).

Bernard's experimentation was recapitulated several decades later at the University of Toronto, where Professor John McLeod did extensive work on the pancreas and gallstones. Frederick Banting, a young member of his staff, was interested in the search for a treatment for diabetes, and McLeod gave him the facilities to pursue his work (43). In 1921, Banting and his medical student, Charles Best, injected a crude pancreatic extract into the buttocks of Leonard Thompson, a frail 14-year-old boy with severe diabetes. The boy's blood sugar levels came down, but he developed serious infections in both hips. Banting and Best thereupon enlisted James Collip to purify the extract. Six weeks later, Thompson was given another preparation with a purer insulin content. The results were amazing. His blood sugar level fell from 522 to 120 in 24 hours. His strength and weight quickly improved, and he lived well until he died of pneumonia at age 27.

Elsewhere, Frederick Allen, who was heralded as the leading American diabetic expert of the early 20th century, was suggesting that since the diabetic's body could not handle food very well and sugar in particular, some hope might be derived from restricting calorie consumption (44). His starvation treatment was labeled bizarre and cruel, but since no one had anything better to offer, patients flocked to his New Jersey office for the regimen. Since there was at the time no understanding of the different types of diabetes, some of his patients improved, while others died.

One of Allen's most famous patients was Elizabeth Evans Hughes, daughter of Charles Evans Hughes, then governor of New York and eventually chief jus-tice of the U.S. Supreme Court. Elizabeth had severe diabetes. In desperation, she consulted Allen and his team, who reduced her calories to 400 per day. She called it a nightmare. After years in Allen's care, she consulted Banting in

August 1922. She weighed 45 pounds, was unable to walk, and was scarcely alive. Banting started her on insulin and then a higher-calorie diet, and she became stronger and began to thrive. Elizabeth lived a long, happy, and productive life, and she considered Banting her medical hero.

Banting and his remarkable shot exploded onto the world stage. MacLeod and Banting won the Nobel Prize in Medicine in 1923. Banting shared his award with Best, while MacLeod shared his with Collip. Fabled diabetes disease expert Elliot P. Joslin, who went on to start the world-famous Joslin Clinic, published a medical paper in 1948 in which he reported that the pre-insulin additional life expectancy of a 6-year-old with diabetes was 1.3 years, of a 30-year-old 4.1 years, and a 50-year-old 8 years (45). After insulin, in 1948, the 6-year-old had a future life expectancy of 67 years, the 30-year-old had 31 more years, and the 50-year-old had 16 more years. The insulin miracle, one of the first truly legitimate medical treatments, was confirmed over and over.

## The Modern Era: The Age of Wonder Drugs and Genes

The improved nutrition and sanitation that preceded Pasteur's magnificent discovery had blunted the viciousness of infectious disease epidemics. Yet it was not until 1935 that Gerhard Domagk, director of research for I.G. Farbenindustrie in Germany, published a seminal report on the sulfa drug Prontosil Red, a commercial dye that had been used for coloring textiles (46). In 1932, Domagk found that when he gave Prontosil to mice that had been injected with lethal doses of hemolytic Streptococcus, they recovered. Streptococci had been known to be the causes of scarlet fever, strep throat, rheumatic fever, erysipelas, and puerperal fever, but there had been no effective treatment against them. Domagk successfully treated his own daughter for a strep infection with his new compound, but it was not until sulfa saved the life of Winston Churchill, who was seriously ill with pneumonia at a critical stage of World War II, that the miracle drug achieved appropriate recognition. Domagk was awarded the Nobel Prize in 1939, but Hitler's Gestapo prevented him from accepting it. He was finally able to do so in 1947.

The fact that a chemical compound was so gloriously successful in combating one of the cruelest scourges was the intellectual spark that quickly led to Florey and Fleming's discovery of penicillin (47). The production of penicillin in 1940 represented a major advance over the sulfa compounds, which only restrained the growth of bacteria but did not kill them, as penicillin did.

The discoveries of sulfa, penicillin, and insulin gave medicine its first real science-based credentials. From then on, medical teaching had something to teach, and medical practice had legitimate therapy to offer. This ignition point, the lift-off that Medicine had awaited since humankind was born, was attained only a cosmic nanosecond ago.

Our ability to heed the Oracle's commandment to know ourselves has been dramatically increased by our recent exploration of life at the molecular level. Merely examining our surface contours did not yield much of value to Medicine. Now we have a virtual anatomic atlas of ourselves at an atomic level. But such structural knowledge leaves begging the larger issues of how we function and how we came to be. There simply is no bigger question in human biology than "How do we happen?" What, and where, is the design manual?

The notion of heredity, even in the case of diseases, has been the subject of speculation since antiquity. Modern genetics was jump-started by the experiments of the Bohemian monk Gregor Mendel, who conducted elaborate cross-breeding experiments with the common garden pea. His work, first presented in 1865, lay fallow until it was discovered that the cell's nucleus, where the cell's heredity machinery was thought to reside, contains a substance, labeled nucleic acid, of two varieties, DNA and RNA.

It remained, however, for Frances Crick and Thomas Watson to elaborate on the physical structure of the nucleic acids in 1953 (48). Their mapping of the now-famous double helix explained the mechanism of genetics. The clinical payoff from this breakthrough was immense and instantaneous. Medical science was vastly enriched by this new way of seeing what had previously been obscure, and these early pioneers were granted rock star status.

The possibility of commercial exploitation of this new knowledge led immediately to the expansion of the biotech industries. Gene transplantation became a reasonable forecast. The Stanford Medical Center Department of Biochemistry is one of the mother churches of gene technology, where several Nobel Prizes are displayed. The campus was virtually trembling with excitement at the Human Genome Project begun in 1990, a Manhattan Project-style effort that sought to decode the entire 30,000-plus genes of our species' nature. The day of revelation came in April 2003. Three-inch headlines proclaimed the occasion, and television satellite trucks swarmed the campus.

At 4 p.m., one of Stanford's Nobel laureates, Arthur Kornberg, delivered the celebratory speech to mark the occasion. Fairchild Auditorium was standing room only as he began: "Ladies and gentlemen, we assemble here today to recognize one of mankind's greatest achievements, the unraveling of the human genome. With this new capacity we will soon be able to rid mankind of most of its scourges and sorrows. We now can go to the bookstore and purchase a rendering of our most intimate selves." Waves of applause met his remarks (49).

## Medical Education and Research

Though we have leafed through thousands of years of medical history, we have not made much mention of medical education, which is such an important component of the structure of Current Medicine. That is because most of history produced no sturdy blocks of knowledge to build upon. Apart from some crude centers of learning in Arabia, China, India, Alexandria, and Edinburgh, medical education for centuries consisted chiefly of an ad hoc apprenticeship arrangement. Eventually, a knowledge of Latin and some courses in philosophy were required for entry into the field. Later still, some college attendance was preferred. But in 1910, my Uncle Walter entered Jefferson Medical School in Philadelphia directly after graduating from Greensburg High School. And in those days, med graduates went straight from school into medical practice, as Uncle Walter did. It was not until the 1920s that postdoctoral training, consisting of internship, residency, and fellowship, was added.

In the mid-19th century, the American medical education system was probably the worst in the industrial world. It was beset by villainy and jealousies, but predominantly by venality. Two comments by Charles Eliot, who became president of Harvard in 1861, summed up the state of Harvard Medical School at that time. In his presidential report of 1869, he called the school "a money-making institution, not much better than a diploma mill" (50). And in 1871, he remarked, "The ignorance and general incompetency of the average American medical graduate at the time when he receives the degree which turns him loose upon the community is something horrible to contemplate" (51). In 1854 Abraham Lincoln pleaded and succeeded in the application to the Illinois state legislature of the first school of homeopathy for credentialing (52).

### Setting Up a New Model

In 1878, William Welsh returned from his studies in Germany to Johns Hopkins University, where a momentous development was to occur with the founding of the Johns Hopkins Medical School. It represented a new model: it was to be a 4-year medical school with full course components, examinations, laboratories, clinical clerkships, and all the other features that constitute what we now consider to be a developed school. Welsh and William Osler set the standard at Johns Hopkins that the other leading medical schools would follow. Hopkins drew immediate financial support from the community.

Many years later, in 1908, Abraham Flexner, a young founder and director of a progressive college preparatory school, issued an appraisal of American educational institutions, after which the Carnegie Foundation commissioned him to report on the state of American medical education. He and the AMA Council on Medical Education collaborated to produce the famous Flexner Report of 1910, which is considered by some to be the most important document in the history of American medicine (53). It was a scathing report, incriminating faculty, facilities, and operations. It also recommended a standardized medical school curriculum of 2 years of basic science followed by 2 years of clinical training.

Flexner hoped that his report would strengthen the strong schools and liquidate the rest. And in fact, 91 schools were driven out of business. Of the 162 "schools" of 1906 there remained 131 in 1910 and 81 in 1922. Flexner hoped to winnow them down to only 31, but after his report, 71 remained.

Before the Flexner Report, there were seven medical schools for black students. Today, only Howard and Meharry remain. Flexner's recommended changes cost money, and the black medical schools had less access to funding than their white counterparts. Some have said that the report was also particularly harsh in criticizing the black schools and their faculty, making it hard for most of the schools to attract good students and stay in business.

In fact, the improvements suggested in the Flexner Report were so expensive that they hastened an exodus from the medical-education business. The clinical clerkship replaced the traditional didactic lecture representing the chief mode of teaching, having the students learn by doing instead of listening. This development was tremendously human-capital intensive. But the "see one, do one, teach one" method proved resilient, even if it depended on a role-model system that varied with the teaching skills of the role model.

### The Founding and Rise of the AMA

Recognizing the tumult that was taking place in the medical marketplace in the middle of the 19th century, a small group of doctors in New York City got together and formed the American Medical Association (AMA) in 1847, mostly to solidify credentialing practices. At the tender age of 30, Dr. Nathan Smith Davis had offered a resolution during a meeting of the New York

Medical Association suggesting that a national medical association was needed "to elevate the standards of medical education in the United States" (54). Dr. Nathaniel Chapman, the first president of the AMA, told the 1848 convention in Baltimore that "the profession to which we belong, once venerated on account of its antiquity, its varied and profound science, its elegant literature, its polite accomplishments, its virtues—has become corrupt and degenerate to the forfeiture of its social position. Are you not imperatively instructed to purify its taints and abuses and restore it to its former elevation and dignity?" (55).

The early AMA struggled with legitimacy and survival. It was in open conflict with the nation's marginal medical schools, diploma mills, and the thousands of untrained doctors who posed perhaps the single greatest hazard to the nation's health. In 1881, to address its dire financial state, it decided to finance itself by publishing a scientific weekly, the *Journal of the American Medical Association* (*JAMA*). The same Nathan Smith Davis became its first editor. The journal debuted on July 14, 1883, with a press run of 3,500 copies and a subscription rate of $5 a year.

The AMA remained in turmoil until the early 20th century. In 1904, it created the Council on Medical Education to attempt to apply some order to the medical school chaos. Over the next few years, the Council evaluated the nation's schools three times, and *JAMA* published the results. The big breakthrough came in 1910, when it joined with the Carnegie Foundation to initiate an intensive review of medical education that resulted in the Flexner Report. Under Dr. Arthur Dean Bevan, professor of surgery at the University of Chicago's Rush Medical School, the AMA Council on Medical Education and Hospitals led the struggle to smash the diploma mills, improve medical training, and standardize state medical licensure. So, the Flexner Report came after a great deal of work done by the Council on Medical Education, and not before it.

As a result of the changes demanded by the Flexner Report, and the increasing strength of the AMA's dedication to higher medical education training standards, American medical school education transformed itself. Whereas in 1860 it was alleged that American schools were the worst in the world, by 1920 they were the best (56).

At the time of World War I, the AMA and its constituent societies had gained unchallenged authority in all fields of health. State health agencies relied on the state medical societies. Standards were set by both as they began the task of sanctioning hospitals to train new physicians. The AMA became the authoritative source of advice on training of nurses and technicians.

*Crunching the Numbers: Med Schools Tie to Hospitals
and Universities*

The business side of medical education began to reflect a trend common to many businesses: to get better, they needed to get bigger. But they started small. In 1891, the Yale Medical School's endowment was $500,000, compared to the Divinity School's $18 million (57). The average medical school yearly operating budget in 1900 was $100,000. By 1910, virtually all U.S. medical schools were self-sufficient financially. And medical school faculty salaries were under control: in 1931 they ranged from $1,000 to $16,000 a year. Paul Beeson, one of the patriarchs of American medicine when he was professor at Yale Medical School in 1952, made $18,000 annually.

Since just before World War II, however, medical school budgets have grown exponentially. By 1940, the average medical school's yearly operating budget was $1 million. By 1960, it was $52 million a year, and by 1990 $200 million a year. Many schools were much larger. As the 20th century wore on, medical schools addressed their growing capital needs by several means: community philanthropic support, which grew when the medical school was viewed as a worthy community resource; formally allying with hospitals; and becoming actively involved in funded research.

Academic medical centers came into being. By definition, an academic medical center has three components: a medical school, a hospital (or clinic), and a research center. The establishment of this three-part structure set off many chain reactions that changed medicine forever. For example, the association of the medical school with a hospital and its large array of technical support gave a tremendous boost to the growth of modern surgery. When virulent bacteria were finally brought under control, surgical medicine began to thrive. The highly theatrical nature of surgery led to a higher fee schedule. People simply valued the services supplied by the cutting doctors more than they did those of the thinking doctors, and surgeons started making more money.

In her book about the flowering of the Mayo Clinic, Helen Clapesattle recorded that the founders, Will and Charlie Mayo, had performed 54 abdominal operations between 1889 and 1892 (58). This total swelled to 612 in 1900 and 2,157 in 1905. Will Mayo published an article in a surgical journal describing the results of 1,000 gallbladder operations he had performed. The early clinics—Mayo, Lahey, Cleveland (Crile), and Ochsner—were all led by surgeons, with their strong financial statements. This surgical bonanza provided the medical schools with another way of paying the salaries of their non-surgical faculty: they simply subsidized the lower earners.

Meanwhile, the non-surgeons were being encouraged to help pay for part of their salaries by fees for patient care. This arrangement caused two problems. First, it created a town–gown schism, as the local practitioners competed for the same patient base as the medical faculty members, but without the gloss of the university affiliation. As the medical schools and their academic medical centers grew in prominence and prestige, there was increasing contention between the town and gown. Second, requiring the faculty to see patients for a wage nominally conflicted with their first obligation, teaching. This dilemma persists today.

Combining the schools with universities and hospitals created institutions that were administratively, professionally, economically, and scientifically superior. A simple, modest cottage industry was in the process of becoming a social, political, and economic behemoth. Paul Starr called the resulting structure "sovereign" (59). Its political muscle was enormous. In the United States, as in all developed countries, it became the largest industry in the land.

### The Rise of Research

Throughout history, science has sought deeper understanding by taking things apart. Our principal research technique goes by the general term of reductionism, taking a thing apart to see what it is made of and how it works. The successes resulting from this dissection approach are apparent everywhere. The relentless pursuit of reductionism has yielded two of the main pillars of modern medicine, the first in the research domain and the second in the realm of medical practice.

The emergence of research has had an enormous influence on medical school faculties. The 20th century provided a steamroller impetus for medical research funded by several sources: local and national philanthropic donations (in 1945 the Rockefeller Foundation was the single largest donor to medical research); government funding, which would eventually total billions of dollars; and finally the drug companies, which found eager partners in the research-minded medical schools. Big Pharma was to become the single largest patron of medical school salaries. But this support came with a heavy price tag.

The ability to recruit and pay faculty came to be largely a matter of who was able to obtain the biggest research grants. The medical school thereby became a research institute first and a teaching institution second. The rise of research in academic medical centers led to a corresponding rise in applied research, and technological breakthroughs followed (60). As Aristotle knew, reason alone is a low-powered beam into the darkness. Expansion of knowledge is intimately associated with tools. For most of history, medicine's instruments had been crude and had provided only scant glimpses into how we are made and how we function. The stethoscope and the thermometer yielded little knowledge of our insides. The microscope and the X-ray made this terra incognita more knowable, but they were developed only a little over 100 years ago.

I was a judge at a large high school science contest sponsored by Intel a few years ago. It featured a dozen Nobel Prize winners who talked about their careers. Ten of the 12 said that they won their Nobels as a direct result of a technological breakthrough that had allowed them to see beyond what others had seen. My humble research career was largely based on the availability of radioactive carbon generated at the Lawrence Radiation Lab in Berkeley. C-14 allowed scientists around the world to track the metabolic pathways involved in our basic carbon substrates. This information led to thousands of original research papers. The research community has enthusiastically exploited the explosion of electronic gadgetry. The computer, above all, has opened up the research frontier, accelerating the pace of developments.

At the frontier of research, a new discipline, known as systems biology, is emerging. Harvard recently created a new department of systems biology, which acknowledges the necessity of putting back together what we waited for so long to take apart. Three years ago, I was among a group of 30 like-minded individuals who put together an international conference at the NIH entitled, "The Dynamic and Energetic Basis of Health and Aging" (61). We sketched the new frontier of self-understanding. Our major recommendation, which we conveyed to the NIH Director, Dr. Elias Zerhouni, was to close the Gene Institute and open the new Institute on Systems Biology. We must confront the issue, "Does the research enterprise serve the patient or the research enterprise?"

# The Practice of Medicine and the | 4
# Rise of the Technological Imperative

After training and research, the third leg of the health care triangle is the actual practice of medicine. The profession has changed dramatically over the past 100 years with the rise of both specialists and technologists and an increasingly business-oriented medical ecosystem.

To know how the profession has changed, we need to remember where it started. In the last paragraph of *The Greatest Benefit to Mankind: A Medical History of Humanity,* Professor Roy Porter wrote, "For centuries medicine was impotent and thus unproblematic. From the Greeks to the First World War its tasks were simple: to grapple with lethal diseases and gross disabilities, and to ensure live births and manage pain. It performed these with meager success" (1). Voltaire said, "Physicians are individuals who prescribe medicines of which they know little, for diseases of which they know less, to persons of whom they know nothing" (2). As we showed in the last chapter, medicine's centuries-long impotence to advance itself explains why descriptions of medical practice are generally absent from the story of human enlightenment. Medicine, through most of its history, lacked a central orthodoxy. It had no organizing framework. The values of professionalism, charity, and samaritanism were often subordinated to those of crass commercialism.

## The Profession's Changing Dynamics

Gradually, population changes began to determine much of the future course of medicine. The U.S. population grew from 250,000 in 1702 to 4 million in 1800 and 80 million in 1900. In 1830, the average practitioner earned about $500, much of it from numerous non-medical tasks such as tending a neighbor's live-stock, pulling teeth, spending the night with a feverish child, or embalming corpses. In 1850, a doctor would see an average of five to seven patients a day. By 1940, that number had grown to 20.

By 1910, doctors were making between $750 and $1,500 per year, about the same as ministers, but less than federal employees. One third of small-town MDs in 1914 had moved to the city and larger-practice opportunities by 1925, largely because of population increases. By then, the typical physician was making about $5,000 yearly, roughly twice the pay of a day laborer. Average physician income fell back to $3,000 per year during the early years of the Depression, but by 1937 pay was up to $3,500 to $7,500 a year.

Another changing dynamic that affected the profession was technology. As early as 1850, the first diagnostic tools—the stethoscope, the laryngoscope, and the ophthalmoscope—increased the physician's competence. The doctor could now "see inside." Within the past 100 years, those tools morphed into X-rays and the electrocardiograph, both of which came into common use to monitor the body's internal functions. These were soon followed by ultrasound, CT scans, and magnetic resonance imaging (MRI). Devices like the hypodermic needle date back to as early as the 1850s, and more sophisticated devices like the pacemaker and artificial heart gave physicians even more to work with.

At the same time, they helped fuel the explosive rise in medical expenses. There has been an exponential increase in technological sophistication. We seem to be hopelessly addicted to technological fixes. And this addiction is not new: when I was in medical school in 1953, the diagnostic workup of an unre-mitting headache would involve a head X-ray, which rarely yielded much of value. The next step was to drill holes in the skull and inject air through a needle into the brain's ventricles—a pneumoencephalogram, a miserable, painful, marginally informative procedure. Now, fortunately, that procedure is only a memory.

We have before us now a variety of brain imaging techniques that display not only the microanatomy of the deep brain structures, but their active func-tioning as well. The field of diagnostic radiology has spawned the major new specialty of interventional radiology, which provides diagnostic and therapeu-tic approaches to previously remote body parts. There is no terra incognita left. All is exposed, but at a huge cost. Virtually every American hospital with over

200 beds has a CT scanner or MRI machine (or two or three). The effect of this machinery on hospital revenues is immense. In 2007, 27.5 million MRI scans were performed, a 3% increase in a year. An article in the *New England Journal of Medicine* reported that there were 62 million CT scans per year, one third of which were deemed unnecessary. This is in contrast to 3 million CT scans in 1980. Note that these are not innocuous procedures (3). An estimated doubling of average personal radiation exposure has occurred nationally as a result of this upsurge in scanning, and it is projected that 2% of cancers in the decades ahead will be attributable to current overuse of the CT scanners. If a 45-year-old has a yearly body scan until age 75, he accumulates a 1 in 50 chance of developing a cancer as a result of this radiation, similar to an atom bomb survivor (4).

In 2007, the CEO of Kaiser, George Halvorson, wrote a book called *Epidemic of Care,* in which he shines a bright light on medicine's love affair with its devices (5). Too many high-tech tests and too many high-tech treatments are evidence that we, both physicians and patients, will go to great lengths to be sure that we have the latest high-powered platinum-coated super-machine at our instant summons. A Stanford Medical Grand Rounds featured a presentation by a colleague who demonstrated that (at trivial added value) a linear accelerator (which we happen to have just up the hill) can provide increased diagnostic competence of heart disease—never mind that its cost would bankrupt certain Third World countries.

As the range of diagnostic competence is vastly increased, so too are the unanticipated consequences. Each progressive miniaturization leads to further uncertainty. Such uncertainty has led to the new term, "incidentaloma." An "oma" is a lump or tumor (carcinoma: cancerous lump; lipoma: fatty lump, etc.). An incidentaloma is a shadow or lump that appears unexpectedly on the X-ray. Its nature is obscure even to the experienced radiologist. When such an incidentaloma occurs, it immediately sparks the need to explain the unexpected finding. The resulting secondary search in turn prompts its own added uncertainties, and so on. Each generation of investigation spurs further expense.

Dr. Barnett Kramer, director of the National Institutes of Health Office of Disease Prevention, said: "For every hundred people who undergo a scan somewhere, between 30 and 80 of them will be told that there is something that needs a workup. And it will likely turn out to be nothing" (4)—an incidentaloma. The American College of Radiology and the FDA have issued similar restraining comments, so the scan-scam has tapered off. This story does not mean that scans are worthless; far from it: they remain one of the most valued of the new medical technologies. Nonetheless, indiscriminant over-scanning remains a significant and dubious cost issue. Figuring out the cost/benefit ratio of this and other tools is crucial—and in this instance "cost" means more than just cash.

But similar to the body scan story, gene-probing technology has its own unexpected consequences, an "incidentalome." This term was coined by Isaac Kohane from the Center for Biomedical Informatics at Harvard and his colleagues in the July 12, 2006, issue of *JAMA* (6). They warn that disastrous consequences may erupt from gene-probing technology. Physicians will be overwhelmed by the complexity of pursuing unexpected genomic measurements and patients will be subjected to unnecessary follow-up tests, causing additional morbidity and anxiety. The chances of spurious results amplify as the number of tests multiply.

The human genome is widely celebrated as the new kid on the science block. Each of us has his or her own personal genome available as an annotated gene array, our entire 21,000-per-cell gene portrait (the estimated number of genes we have is constantly being revised). The expansion of diagnostic and prognostic opportunity brought about by genomic patterns numbs the mind. For a few hundred dollars for a personal genome scan, 300,000 single nucleotide patterns can be measured. This is well recognized by commercial interests that want to send you and your loved ones your personal gene profiles, much in the way of allowing you to name your own personal star in the heavens. The new frontier of "personalized medicine" seeks to institutionalize this commercial opportunity.

But in the real world of clinical medicine, gene pattern analysis is much more complicated than the superficial display might indicate, because it is in the interaction of the genes over time that the real world operates. The presence or absence of a single gene is almost irrelevant. Meanwhile, medical costs skyrocket in pursuit of this sci-fi scenario.

The profession would complete its rise from wretchedness with the help of these technologies and drugs. It now had its first real science-based credentials. From then on, medical practice had legitimate therapy. But there was another dynamo at work in the rise from wretchedness: the AMA.

## The Continuing Role of the AMA: The Profession's Advocate

By the 1920s, Medicine had become more grounded in science (biology and chemistry especially) and more regulated (even if most of that was self-regulation). The AMA had a role in both developments, and insisted that the doctor's relationship with the patient was primary—the patient's well-being came before all else. The AMA became a national voice via its insistence that patients were entitled to the highest possible quality of care. It was influential in passing pure food and drug legislation, exposing unscientific remedies, and stigmatizing cultism and quackery. The AMA achieved recognition as a public benefactor and a model of what could be accomplished through private initiative. It had therefore transformed itself from a tattered group of fringe physicians to the dominant voice in American medicine. It became a trade organization with a principal orientation toward maintaining the autonomy of its members. As a sign of its success, it mushroomed from 8,000 members in 1900 to 70,000 by 1910, representing half of the nation's physicians.

The AMA's Council on Medical Education eventually morphed into the American Board of Medical Specialists. I had my own experience with this group when I was president of the American Geriatrics Society (AGS) in 1981. There was an effort to make geriatrics into a subspecialty of internal medicine, as was the pattern in Great Britain. I felt, however, that geriatrics was too large an area to be sequestered into a minor specialty, and that the aging of the population predicted that all doctors, not a particular few, were destined to take care of old people. After several closed-door hearings the AMA Board took the statesmanlike step of creating an area of special competency for that physician who exhibits a commitment to the care of older patients, notably not endorsing the establishment of another specialty.

Of course, any account of the AMA's influence on the modern profession has to include its reaction to attempts to bring more governmental control and funding into Medicine. My father was president of the AMA in 1947 and was deeply involved in the Medicare transition. The AMA was feverishly opposed to any entry of the government into the financing of health care, fearing control over doctors' incomes. The organization, then as now, was dominated by the surgeons whose incomes were generous and whose practices allowed them time for politicking. The surgeons and their adjacent specialties of anesthesia, pathology, and radiology were the prime players.

The AMA in my father's presidential era appropriated millions of dollars to counteract a perceived flirtation with socialized medicine. The election of Franklin Delano Roosevelt in 1932 represented a major break in social politics as the New Deal gave us Social Security, but there was little initiative for including medical care within this new structure. Roosevelt chose to wait. The next historic moment occurred in 1965, when, as Secretary of Health, Education and Welfare under President Lyndon Johnson, John Gardner ushered in Medicare and Medicaid. These government-sponsored programs, rather than pinching the physician's wallet, eventually became a bonanza, as frequently unreimbursed services became billable. At the same time, the increasing numbers of gray-haired patients achieved a higher level of medical security. We are warned, however, that the massive funding of Medicare and Medicaid now threatens the solvency of our nation.

## The Generalists Become Specialists

As far back as the fifth century BC, Herodotus wrote of the Egyptian practice of training physicians by concentrating on just one part of the body (7). Such early specialization stood in opposition to the Greek insistence that the whole body should be the object of observation. Hippocrates, after all, was a generalist, and so were most physicians for most of medical history.

Early American physicians were representative of the rest of the population in their fierce independence and distrust of government and other forms of institutionalized authority. But a strong current boosting specialization has pushed this major change in the profession over the past century. This force included increased pressure for the hospital to serve as a location for specialized testing and treatment. Gradually, access to operating rooms, X-ray equipment, and other laboratory machinery was confined to those who had an extra-special diploma on their walls. This trend, in turn, begat the biotech industry, with its acres of devices demanding special know-how (8).

The concentration of influence in the hospital instead of the office was strengthened when use of the hospital was restricted to specialists, specifically in Great Britain, as specified in the National Health Service. But this was also sporadically and individually negotiated in the United States, with much distress, alarm, and discomfort. Local private practitioners found their hospital-based privileges progressively constricted by the academic MDs, with immediate, large financial consequences (9).

Specialization arose not as the result of an organized process, but simply by what seemed to work. Some specialization was based on organs, some on diseases, some on gender, some on age. It was not a coincidence that the ophthalmology and otolaryngology specialists became the first two groups to provide certifying exams for their physicians, to separate them from the competition that lacked extra training. Specialization was not confined to physicians, as hospitals also broke down into niche service areas. Our sister vocation of dentistry specialized itself to good effect, as did the veterinarians.

In 1940, 77% of physicians were general practitioners (GPs), but by 1970 that number was down to 30% and falling. The family doctor was becoming an endangered species. A 1968 prediction targeted the year 2000 as the funeral date for general practice. Medical students, obviously affected by the examples and counsel of their specialist professors, ensconced in the ivory towers of the

university teaching hospitals, began to show a marked preference for specialization over generalization.

Specialization has become medicine's dominant agenda. The desire to be an
expert in something is clearly an incentive; so too is the prestige accorded to
someone judged to have a special ability. But without question, the chief reason
is financial. Specialists make more money. The generalist sells time, the specialist
sells technology. Technology is faster, and time is money.

The specialist mentality routinely demeans the competence of the family
doctor. I can recall instances when a patient's care was characterized during
teaching case presentations in medical school sessions as having been provided
by "just a GP," connoting inferior care. Such disparagement impugns the family
practitioner and the GP, who resent hints of condescension and argue justifi-
ably that the family practitioners and GPs represent the last "real doctors"—
idealistic—whose patient is the prime contractor. The GP is quick to remind
the specialist of Osler's famous dictum: "It is not which disease the patient has
which is foremost, it is which patient has the disease" (10).

## The Specialist in an Industrial Setting:
## The Medical-Industrial Complex

Arnold Relman, former editor of the *New England Journal of Medicine*, coined
the term "medical-industrial complex" (MIC) in a 1980 article in that journal (8).
In it, he detailed how the MIC of hospitals, surgery, technology, and pharmacy
has rapidly transformed medicine from a relatively modest cottage industry
into a giant mega-corporation with manifold repercussions. My term for the
MIC is the "disease cartel." Similarly, Paul Starr's central book, *The Social
Transformation of American Medicine*, details the cataclysmic changes that were
invoked in medicine by the flood of new money that was made available chiefly
by the passage of the Medicare law in 1965 (9).

In 1910, Will Mayo declared that medical practice demanded a collective
rather than an individual approach (11). In 1920, driven by the escalation of
medical costs, early insurance protocols were introduced. The importance
of this cannot be overemphasized. For the first time, fee-for-service payment
was transferred to a detached "buy now, pay later" insurance process. This
insulation from personal immediate responsibility for payment has had a
huge impact. In 1932, the Blues insurance programs were initiated. In 1938
Sydney Garfield introduced a novel medical care system at the Grand Coulee
Dam project of the Kaiser Corp. (12). In it the physician became a salaried
employee. Payment in this case was made by the employer up front, in a

prenegotiated arrangement. This abrogation of the time-honored doctor/ patient fee for service was an immediate flashpoint, "defiling the doctor–patient relationship." The great preponderance of physicians whose practice pattern was "fee for service" and their organizational cartel, the AMA, perceived an ominous threat to their precious professional autonomy.

Still, the traditional fee-for-service mechanism of medical finance persisted until the 1970s, when different insurance approaches drew new attention. In 1969, Paul Ellwood and Lou Butler, physician iconoclasts, advised President Richard Nixon, who advocated for some form of prepaid medical coverage. But it was Alain Enthoven, in his 1978 *New England Journal of Medicine* article, who provided the term "managed competition" as a template for medical insurance (13). It added the vital component of "competition" to the generic term "managed care." Whereas Enthoven's formulation has been adopted by several foreign nations in their effort to reconcile the cost–benefit interface, and the Clinton health care misadventure of 1993 mangled the opportunity for its implementation here, the central plank of managed competition remains sturdy.

Adding to the explosive changes wrought by specialization and third-party payers from 1950 onward was the categorical shift in the types of clinical problems that doctors confronted. Throughout history, Medicine had been chiefly concerned with the acute conditions of infection and trauma, in which the illness, diagnosis, treatment, and payment all occur within a short timeframe. In middle of the 20th century, this form of medicine was replaced by an entirely different presentation, that of chronic illness. This is one of the most important changes in medicine, and its effects remain largely unaddressed in terms of allocation of personnel and resources.

It is now reported that 72% of physician visits are due to chronic conditions, as are 76% of hospital admissions. Chronically ill persons use three times as much medical manpower as those with acute illnesses: 7.4 versus 1.7 doctor visits per year. The person who has five or more chronic conditions visits the doctor an average of 15 times a year. Fourteen percent of persons with chronic illness say they never have a good day. Implicit in this structural shift from acute to chronic is the aging of the population. Simply put, more illnesses occur in old people, and when they do, they last longer and cost more.

## The Effects of Change

Any examination of the ecology of Current Medicine has to include two articles in the *New England Journal of Medicine,* one from 1961 and the other from 2001, with the title "The Ecology of Medical Care" (14,15). Their findings, shown in Figure 4.1, offer a helpful framework for thinking about the organization of health care and medical personnel. In any given month, of every 1,000 people in a community, 800 may have symptoms of illness; 200 of those see a doctor and 10 are hospitalized. In my view, the formatting of these reports is even more important than the actual numbers. Important qualitative judgments arise. First, it is clear that using the hospital as a classroom for learning about medicine is a gross misrepresentation of reality. Second, each of the encounter categories, and particularly the interface between them, can be used to project the ideal medical care allotment. Much specific directed effort should apply at each of the interfaces to minimize the tendency to graduate to the next more intensive care zone.

While neither of the above articles presents cost data, it is implicit in both that as the interfaces shift, so too do the costs (Figure 4.2). In other words, the further the arrow points to the left, the more economical the resulting product will be. The further it points to the right, indicating that more is being done, the more expensive the care becomes.

What does our present emphasis on specialty care have to say about this? How much high-tech intensive care is being delivered by underqualified physicians? Not much, I suspect. But the reverse—how much low-tech care is being delivered by overqualified doctors?—is an immense issue about which there

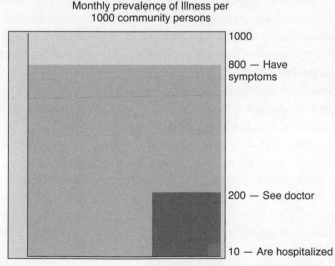

**Figure 4.1** Ecology of medical care. From "The Ecology of Medical Care Revisited," *New England Journal of Medicine*, June 2001, Volume 344, page 2023. Copyright © 2001, Massachusetts Medical Society. All rights reserved.

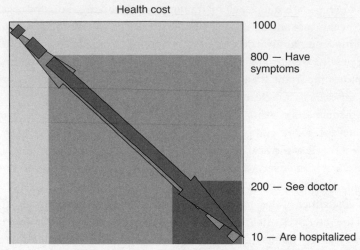

Health cost

1000

800 — Have
symptoms

200 — See doctor

10 — Are hospitalized

**Figure 4.2** Costs of ecology. Green, L.G. Fryer, B. Yawn, D. Lanier, S. Dovey. Ecology of Medical Care Research New England. *Journal of Medicine*, 2001, 344:2021–2025.

has been no extensive discussion. Clayton Christensen, a professor at Harvard Business School, makes a major issue of the "overshoot" of medical competency and need, a mismatch between the actual care required by the patient's problem and the firepower of the medical response (16). Does every twitch in your chest require a multispecialized interventional cardiologist? Does every freckle presume a dermatologist visit? Particularly if this overshoot costs megabucks?

Countless commissions have studied and made recommendations on this score, the most renowned being the Physician Payment Review Commission (PPRC), formerly led by Phil Lee, Assistant Secretary of Health under Presidents Johnson and Clinton. One of the most prejudicial moments comes when the medical student selects a career path. The average medical student, at graduation, is in debt to the tune of somewhere between $50,000 and $100,000. At this fragile moment, which career are you likely to pursue? A medical specialty or general practice?

When I was president of the AGS, I held that one of my chief responsibilities was to do whatever I could to enlist the brightest and best medical students into a career in geriatrics. The need is certainly there. This brought me into direct confrontation with the CEO of the AARP, Cy Brickfield. His lobby maintained a fervent drum beat about physician fees. Any threat, perceived or real, to their pets of Medicare and Medicaid provoked alarm. I presented my case to him, hoping that he might make an exception for geriatrics in his stringency campaign. My pleading fell on deaf ears. "Listen, Walter, I have closets full of testimonials from patients who certify how they have been financially ravaged by you docs," he told me. "We're out to redress this." That was the end of the conversation. I was subsequently able to make my arguments to the elected leadership of the AARP, pointing out that the high rollers, whom he was targeting, are the specialists with high-priced operations and gimmicks that inflate the bill. The geriatricians, I maintained, had no gimmick or surgery, and were paid strictly for their time in making house calls or nursing home visits, which Medicare had decided to reimburse at AARP insistence at the rate of about $30 per hour. How was I to make my arguments to the brightest and best when they faced career opportunities that virtually guaranteed incomes many times higher than those in geriatrics and general practice?

## The Pursuit of Satisfaction and Effectiveness

With all the negative commentary about the glut of specialists and dearth of primary care docs, we need to check the facts. First, are doctors happy? Numerous large surveys, including one from Harvard published in *JAMA* in 2003, indicate a high dissatisfaction rate among physicians and offer their testimony that they would not advise prospective students to enter the medical profession (17). A later report, also from Harvard, confirms the gradual erosion of the professional satisfaction quotient (18).

Are the patients happy? Many argue that the high attendance at nontraditional providers' offices, higher than at standard MDs' offices, reflects patients' sense of disaffection. A telling corollary issue is whether the tasks that all physicians pursue—making people feel better and live longer—are being fulfilled. Our longevity is 30 years better than it was 100 years ago. However, we are now being warned that for the first time in our nation's history, this improvement is likely to reverse. Death rates from heart conditions are down significantly, and cancer deaths are down a little, while infectious diseases are in a headlong retreat. Yet many noted scholars, such as John Knowles, René Dubos, John McKinlay, and Thomas McKeown, have observed that these real improvements are due to factors such as improved sanitation and nutrition and lifestyle changes rather than to actual medical interventions.

In his essay "The Effect of Health Services on Health," Robert Haggerty of the Harvard School of Public Health describes what happens when a village of a "primitive" society confronts the medical world (19). Neville Scrimshaw, also at Harvard, and coworkers selected three similar Guatemalan villages; one received modern medicine, the second got medical care plus access to better nutrition, and the third got neither (20). After 5 years, there was hardly any

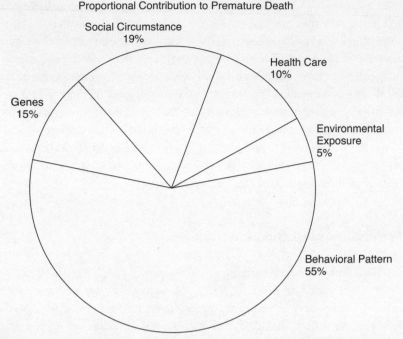

Proportional Contribution to Premature Death

Social Circumstance 19%

Health Care 10%

Genes 15%

Environmental Exposure 5%

Behavioral Pattern 55%

**Figure 4.3** Contribution to premature death. From "We Can Do Better—Improving the Health of the American People," *New England Journal of Medicine*, September 2007, Volume 357, page 1222. Copyright © 2007, Massachusetts Medical Society. All rights reserved.

difference in outcomes except that the preschool children in the first village had more episodes of illness. Similarly, in 1972 Walsh McDermott and colleagues from Cornell Medical College provided modern medical care to 2,000 Navajo Indians living in poverty. "The delivery of this carefully organized and well received primary health care system to Many Farms Community had relatively little influence on disease incidence here," the authors wrote (21).

A third study, the 1970 Welfare Medical Study in New York, showed no difference in morbidity or mortality among aged subjects, even though some received elegant health care at New York Hospital and others received the traditional scattered, disjointed, fragmented care in the community (22). Haggerty concluded, "From these and other evidences what we doctors do for people is rather insignificant" (19).

George Annas, William Fairfield Warren Distinguished Professor and Chair of the Department of Health Law, Bioethics & Human Rights at Boston University School of Public Health, assessed our overall performance: "We do more and more to fewer and fewer people, at higher and higher cost with less and less benefit" (23).

The tectonic changes that describe the rapid evolutionary developments in medical education, research, and practice are reflected in the social and economic realms as well. The science of medicine exhibits a political context that shaped and was shaped by the growth in knowledge and competence.

It is now time to leave Current Medicine's symptoms and long history and propose its diagnosis and treatment.

# Diagnosing Current Medicine | 5

Having reviewed the history, done a basic physical exam, and studied some of the laboratory aspects of the sick patient, Current Medicine, we must now make a diagnosis. I propose that the major entry on the front page of this patient's body chart is total body pain, and the underlying cause is a mismatch between the basic forces of human biology and capitalism. The diagnosis derives directly from the collision between our nature, the biological process that has been deeded to us by millions of years of evolution, and our nurture, our cultural construct of capitalism. As they are currently constituted, these two do not match up and any effort to join them is like trying to jam a square peg into a round hole. A chisel or a hammer or grease will not make it work.

Capitalism is the social contract that most of the world has chosen because it seems to be the best solution to our functional needs (1). It should also fulfill our biological needs. The past five decades have defined these needs as repair and cure, and thereby defaulted on the first principle of health preservation. Current Medicine has been allocated massive resources, while capitalism disserves humankind by endorsing and rewarding illness rather than health. But capitalism itself is not the problem. The problem resides in the product that capitalism has been chosen to sell. Perversely, it peddles dysfunction, disease, and illness. Current Medicine focuses on parts and events, episodes and components. It needs to look at whole processes and systems.

We have seen the historical backdrop of this mismatch. The bedraggled, disease-ridden world was ripe for salvation when Pasteur and the sanitary movement effectively wiped the slate clean of epidemics and their high mortality rates. The world exulted. Doctors were not as incompetent as had been feared. In fact, they routinely delivered miracles on a daily basis. How can we reward them enough? We have done that with billions upon billions of dollars that overnight transformed a sleepy cottage industry into the nation's largest corporation, the Illness Industry. This misshapen dysfunctional entity came into being because the competence of the acute infectious disease era, in which glorious cure was an expected result, was found to be largely impotent when faced with an altered set of conditions.

We are caught in what the sociologists John and Matilda Riley termed "structural lag" (2). This helpful term describes mismatches between change-resistant social structures and "optimal" practices. It applies to a time lag between a substantial cultural event such as the baby boom and the development of the appropriate administrative and economic support systems, schools, and housing. Current Medicine is now in this kind of time warp. We face the new landscape ineffectually, with a worn-out and often perverse system trying to address the new realities with the old tools. Current Medicine is a giant anachronism.

We often seem to be living up to the old social psychology adage that says that when people face a tough and complicated problem, they would rather do nothing than something, because a bad outcome seems more threatening than letting the problem get slowly worse. Bad decisions cause more regret than no decisions, and there is always the chance that the problem will disappear on its own. In the case of Current Medicine's sickness, doing nothing is the worst kind of negligence.

Some have proposed that medicine is in its fatal last swoon, in critical condition. They suggest "do not resuscitate" orders, that it be allowed to die a natural death. Do not bother to thump the chest, it is too late for that. Thumping might restore a heartbeat or two, but it is futile to think that CPR can resolve this catastrophe.

But medicine cannot die. It must survive. To restore it to its primary mission, asserting and assuring human potential, we need to be in a totally different place from where we are now. Our nurture must serve our nature. We have already come a long way: the Fate of prior history, our past ignorance, is now replaced by Choice. Further, our new science allows us to establish a health protocol.

In 2000, while attending the Sydney Olympic Games, my wife and I took a side trip to Alice Springs, a town in the heart of the Australian outback. I paid a courtesy visit to the local health office on Main Street. "How are things going?" I asked the fellow in charge.

"Terrible," he replied. "We are going broke."

"That's not possible," I said, stunned. "Health departments do not go belly up."

He explained. "For 40,000 years, the aborigines have been living half-naked under the stars and walking about. We officials in town said that's not civilized. Come into town and we will take care of you, we told them."

Accordingly, the aborigines came into Alice Springs, found the liquor store, fast-food outlets, and TV, and quickly fell into a sedentary lifestyle and became fat. Diabetes soon followed. Renal failure became commonplace. Many are now on dialysis at $40,000 per person per year. To address this, Dr. Karin O'Dea of Melbourne arranged to relocate a number of aborigines back into the outback, where they began to resume their active lifestyles and normal diet (3). Their diabetes remitted, just as did that of former Arkansas governor Mike Huckabee after he lost weight and embraced marathon running.

We all want to believe that medicine is firmly based on reality, that research systematically identifies important problems and that information is easily transmitted to doctors who apply it unerringly. Unfortunately, the truth is that the practice of Medicine is not based firmly on reality, that the transmission of research information into practice is precarious, and that the results are too often used selectively by practitioners.

The authoritative *Dartmouth Atlas of Health Care* notes, "Spending continues to increase without evidence that what we're doing results in either better outcomes or better patient satisfaction" (4). Author John Wennberg concludes, "The solution for unwarranted variation in preference-sensitive services is shared decision-making, the active involvement of the patient in choosing. Numerous clinical trials have shown that the patient decision-support programs result in better decisions, and often a reduction in utilization. But implementation isn't easy. We need to find a way to encourage and compensate physicians for the time they spend on educating and discussing things with patients."

An efficient system has tools and people that mutually fit its goals, that provide smooth functioning. In the July 27, 2005, issue of *JAMA*, Andy Grove of Intel fame observed that if the computer industry had been saddled with the inefficiencies inherent in the medical system, it would still be back in the hand-crank era (5). For instance, the errors introduced by the paper and phone systems that medicine employs are in the millions. Lives are lost because of insufficient or ignorant use of the Internet. There is a widespread call for standardized automation of medical records. What exists now is too often a smattering of handwritten illegible notations with idiosyncratic, non-standardized comments. I have contributed more than my share of these.

The medical system has millions of employees, 700,000 of whom are physicians. But this number is trivial compared to the support crew. The term "fragmented" understates the situation in the American medical system. It is a patchwork of poorly connected workers laboring in a hodgepodge of non-systems. There are more than 600 insurance companies vying for your business, each with a different format and philosophy. For every physician at a 300-bed hospital in Bellingham, Washington, there are 42 billing clerks. In Vancouver, Canada, on the other hand, there is one billing clerk for a 300-bed hospital (6).

The valuable book *Critical Condition* provides an interesting analogy. The authors, investigative journalists Donald Bartlett and James Steele, reflect on the immense undertaking of the D-Day landings in Normandy (7). What if each of the innumerable battle groups had had its own individual battle plan? It is easy to imagine the total chaos and disaster that would have eventually doomed all the participants. Certainly there were snafus, but generally, considering the vastness of the enterprise, the coordinated effort came off brilliantly.

As I have argued, a major feature of the landscape of American medicine is its emphasis on specialization over generalization. This specialization increases the coefficient of inefficiency in Current Medicine. Whereas other advanced countries display a 20% to 80% ratio of specialists to generalists, the ratio in the United States is 60% to 40%. Unquestionably part of this is due to the exploding science base, which makes it increasingly impossible to master even a proportion of the relevant material. But the financial motive behind specialization is at least as potent an influence. Surgeons earn upwards of $300,000 per year, board-certified internists $240,000, and family practice generalists $144,000. In 1940, there were 37,000 specialists, and today there are more than 400,000. There is a consensus that we need a massive reallocation of physicians from the specialist to the generalist. From a high of 80% of doctors pursuing careers in general practice, the number now is less than 15%. The entire medical training arena is dominated by specialists who naturally tend to replicate themselves and turn out clones who keep the reductionist process going.

## Irrelevance to Relevance

As we consider one of medicine's major symptoms, irrelevance, the question arises: Does medicine have the right people on board, and is it selling the right item? I have used the analogy of the neighborhood on fire, with flames everywhere, sirens screeching, red lights flashing, chaos, and panic. The fire department is professionally trained and has experts in the finest minutiae about the nature of fire. They have the fanciest and most expensive equipment, but they are not very organized, and are rushing madly hither and yon while the situation grows worse. Fires are erupting faster than they are able to get to them. What to do?

Someone suggests that there might be an arsonist at work, and that he or she is cleverer and faster than all the fire departments put together. What the fire departments need is a sleuth instead of a fire chief. They have the wrong personnel for the task at hand. Is this true of Current Medicine?

The second consideration is: Does Current Medicine stock the right goods? It is commonly said that the business of America is business, and business thrives by selling products. But what if medicine is selling the wrong item? What if it is selling shoes, when the public needs textbooks? What if it is selling disease, when the public needs health?

Psychologists often refer to task-relevant and task-irrelevant behavior. If and when Medicine engages fully in the task-relevant behavior of assuring human potential, many of its symptoms begin to go away. One way to assure task-irrelevant behavior is to focus on taking control away from people, replacing the natural with the artificial, and concentrating on technical domination. In his book *The Enigma of Health*, the German philosopher Hans Georg Godamer commented: "Among all the sciences concerned with nature, the science of medicine is the one which can never be understood entirely as a technology, precisely because it invariably experiences its own abilities and skills simply as a restoration of what belongs to nature" (8).

In his book *Limits to Medicine*, the Austrian philosopher and social critic Ivan Illich upbraided medicine for usurping the condition of health for its own purposes (9). Illich takes Current Medicine's irrelevance to our collective health one step further: he argues that it is counterproductive in exactly the same way that traffic jams are counterproductive to effective transportation. Irrelevance implies a disconnect, but counterproductivity implies that Current Medicine is actively opposed to our collective health. In the 2010 State of the World, Transforming Cultures publication I wrote an essay "Reinventing Health Care from Panacea to Hygeia" which reflects the same orientation.

Much as the medieval church used the threat of sin-induced plague to control people's behavior for its own purposes, so Current Medicine presumes to co-opt our own health. The Church reformed itself, but given the pervasiveness of medicine's symptoms, reformation does not seem to be a strong enough solution to the incompatibility between human biology and capitalism. That demands a revolutionary solution.

All of the political solutions being bandied about represent only administrative fixes, mere Band-Aids. What is required is structural change, an approach to the whole as opposed to symptoms. Yes, we need a proper response to achieve cost, equality, safety, transparency, efficiency, and relevance, but this should be provided by structural redress rather than administrative tinkering. Capitalism should serve our health needs, not, as is currently the case, the other way around.

Next Medicine: The Assertion | II
and Assurance of Human
Potential

# Current Medicine's Treatment: Next Medicine | 6

The intersection of breathtaking opportunity and insoluble problem at which we now find ourselves demands a revolutionary response. Once upon a time, Thomas Jefferson wrote, "When in the course of human events it becomes necessary for the people" to challenge and change the ruling position, it is imperative that voices be raised in revolt (1). Our Declaration of Independence recognized that "mankind is more disposed to suffer than to right themselves by abolishing the forces to which they are accustomed," and the practices "long established should not be changed for light and transient causes." But self-evident truths require new goals to effect safety and happiness. William James said, "Great emergencies and crises show us how much greater our vital resources are than we had supposed" (2).

I reference Thomas Kuhn, the noted historian of science from the University of Chicago (3). His 1962 book *The Structure of Scientific Revolutions* stands as one of the landmark insights of the modern era. Kuhn ended his career as professor emeritus of linguistics and philosophy at the Massachusetts Institute of Technology. His earlier life involved studies at the University of California Berkeley, and at the Center for Advanced Study in the Behavioral Sciences at Stanford, where he incubated his catalytic ideas. Kuhn credited James B. Conant, president of Harvard from 1933 to 1953, for his introduction to the history of science that transformed Kuhn's concept of the nature of scientific advance.

Like Paul Romer, he welcomed crisis because it provides the opportunity for a retooling, a resolution of incompatibilities.

Simply stated, Kuhn's rule is that in order to replace a current ruling paradigm that is clearly deficient, a revolution is necessary. Such a revolution has two prerequisites. First, there must be a consensus among the concerned parties that a revolution is required. Massachusetts, Virginia, and the other colonies had to be of a single mind. Second, it is not sufficient merely to demolish the ruling paradigm, but a replacement of sufficient relevance, rigor, and power must be available to substitute for the failed model. Our forefathers crafted a democracy to replace the failed monarchy.

We hold this truth to be self-evident. Kuhn's precept informs and predicts. It asserts that the emergence of a new theory is generally preceded by a pronounced professional insecurity, a sense of malfunction, a major anomaly. That insecurity is generated by the persistent failure of the puzzles of normal science, or politics, to come out as they should. Failure of existing rules is the prelude to a search for new ones.

Kuhn's tenets precisely fit medicine's present circumstance. A new rigorous alternative is required, a new paradigm, whose truth is self-evident and more complete than the former paradigm. We have described the former (and current) paradigm. It is not cost-effective, fair, safe, honest, efficient, or relevant. We have identified its massive shortfall in carrying out medicine's mission of asserting and assuring human potential.

Asserting our human potential is not the hard part of the mission. For the first time in human history, we have a clear view of what a whole human life can look like. Our potential stands revealed for the first time, a gift that is worthy of a hundred Nobel Prizes. None of the prior 151 billion of us has known what he or she was capable of. Now we know the space, span, and pace of our potential. This is an incandescent moment in human history. Medicine has provided an explicit answer to the ignorance and groping of prior history. The human being is a masterpiece of nature's design. Our near perfection is no random accident or metaphysical gift, but the result of relentless surveillance and engineering by our adaptive capabilities. It includes an extraordinary self-repair capacity. I argue that, barring certain circumstances, 100 healthy, fully functional years is each human's potential. The empowerment generated by this new competence in asserting our potential cannot be overestimated.

## A New Paradigm: Next Medicine and Hygeia

To assure rather than merely assert the human potential requires a new paradigm, one that is born out of a return to first principles. We know that

2,500 years ago the Greeks identified that medicine has twin components— Hygeia and Panacea, or health preservation and repair respectively. Of these, Hygeia originally held precedence. The twin functions of medicine survive but are obscured by Panacea's dominance. We have seen that Panacea as Medicine's favored child does not fully assure the human potential. Panacea's elaborate repair capacities are brilliant. But are they fully relevant? Its repair tools of surgery and pharmacy do not fully match our mission statement.

The new paradigm, simply stated, is Next Medicine, the re-introduction of Hygeia into our lives so that Disease Medicine and Health Medicine rebalance themselves and assure our human potential. This involves both health preservation and repair.

Plato's note that life without health is not worth living inserts a high priority for health creation and maintenance. "Every practitioner of medicine needs to be skilled in nature" (4). Next Medicine presides over the total recommitment to the precious first principles that the Greeks declared a long time ago. The validity of the Greek philosophy derived from biological facts of which they knew little, but presumed greatly and wisely.

In medicine's grand embrace of repair and cure, and the huge financial rewards inherent therein, it has defaulted on the maintenance or prevention aspects that make up the essence of health. When Disease Medicine and its counterpart Health Medicine become alloyed, the new broader paradigm, Next Medicine, evolves to fulfill medicine's mission.

Necessity is the mother of invention. What medicine needs today is a new construct: Next Medicine, a medicine that embraces health maintenance (which I have termed Health Medicine) as well as repair and cure. Next Medicine emphasizes self-efficacy and individual responsibility and insists on studying the total organism over time. It asserts that controlling and maintaining health resides primarily with the individual.


## Beyond Healing

Healing is necessary, and for the physician, the healer tradition remains. But it does not define the physician's entire mission. He or she must also assume the additional mantle of teacher. Beyond healing is teaching. This idea suffuses Next Medicine.

It also represents a challenge in the face of the old adage known as Zimmerman's law: "Nobody notices when things go right." Humans typically want instant gratification, whereas prevention strategies play out over time. Further, in a June 20, 2009, *Wall Street Journal* article, "The Myth of Prevention," Professor Abraham Verghese wisely observes that a concise preventive strategy is confounded by its imprecise terminology (5). In his response to President Barack Obama's address to the AMA (6), he correctly shows that if prevention means the extending of expensive high-tech diagnostic efforts to early detection of disease in well people, then the beneficiaries will be the corporate sponsors, not the individual. If, on the other hand, prevention means invoking the core, first principles of health, then the cost/benefit calculus is huge. Inasmuch as most chronic illnesses derive from behavior, a technical focus is unlikely to be of much value. This is particularly evident in the array of income-generating tests that are paraded by the tech and drug people as early detection. These merchandisers promote disease or its threat, which feeds on our innate health anxieties. Most of these are shell games masquerading as early detection or prevention. Prevention is the key, but it must be framed in the appropriate context of self-care. Hippocrates got it right: "Protecting and developing health must rank even above that of restoring it when it is impaired" (7).

In building the case for increased investment in preventive strategies, we must show clearly that it is not only more rational but also cheaper to be healthy now than it is to be sick later. Many reports show that prevention offers a substantial return on investment. There are myriad testimonials from industry reporting reduced absenteeism and reduced disability and health care costs. Yet these reports have not generated a chorus of support for the preventive path. The long timeline inherent in the implementation of preventive strategies is an obstacle in our instant-gratification world.

Figure 6.1, adapted from similar presentations by McGinnis and Foege (8) and Schroeder (9), shows the factors that contribute to premature death. McGinnis and Foege's signal 1993 paper in *JAMA*, "Actual Causes of Death," implicitly says that the principal problems of medicine are not what appears on the death certificate—heart disease, cancer, stroke, and so on—but the ultimate agencies of what I term intrinsic or maintenance medicine. The actual causes of death are not susceptible to the tools of Disease Medicine. Surgical or pharmaceutical approaches cannot address them. Heart attacks, strokes, emphysema, arthritis, and diabetes are not curable, but they are preventable.

The dominance of behavioral causes in the McGinnis and Foege report is profoundly important. If behavior is the "actual" cause of death and illness, then behavioral strategies must be invoked. Medicine has not been active in pursuing such strategies, preferring to embrace what amounts to external therapies for internal problems. But we have to stop defaulting to the repair shop.

Our past confidence in Panacea's competence lessened our reliance on self-care. "Take care of myself" became "Take care of me." We transferred control for our well-being to the medical-industrial complex and came to expect that cure would be the product of Current Medicine's benevolent intercession. Repair was codified as the principal job description of Current Medicine. We need to wake up and pay attention, and assure our potential.

The esteemed microbiologist René Dubos reminds us of what the Greeks saw a long time ago: *Vis medicatrix naturae*, that health is the natural order of things (10). Next Medicine looks again to Hippocrates and restates the age-old philosophy of health that the Greeks embraced. The physician's prime role is to ensure the balance of health, the harmony of the body—not too little, not too much—in concert with the Golden Mean.

"Solving the problems of disease is not the same as creating health and happiness," Dubos wrote in 1979. "This task demands a kind of wisdom and vision which transcends specialized knowledge of remedies and treatments, and which apprehends in all their complexities and subtleties, the relation between living beings and their whole environment." In his call for a Hellenic revival, Dubos notes that human affairs have become medicalized. He rejects the complaint that any effort to limit medicine's reach constitutes recidivism or a denial of science's value. Instead he asserts the need to broaden medicine to include more traditional non-medical areas.

## The Broader Context of Next Medicine

In insisting on a broader context for Next Medicine, we recognize its core elements: the individual, the profession, and society. These are the resources we draw on to achieve our potential, and they must all work together to achieve the greatest good for the greatest number.

For the individual, the focal points are self-efficacy and individual responsibility. For the profession, the new emphasis must be on reassessing its mission, and reallocating personnel and resources. For society and the civic arena in which Next Medicine will operate, the new direction must be toward a larger embrace of community, of collective responsibility.

In contemplating the interrelationship of the three, I am reminded of W. Edwards Deming (11). Deming was the industrial consultant credited with the Japanese miracle. After World War II, he undertook to reshape the entire Japanese industrial sector, which had lapsed into disrepair and inefficiency. He faced an inbred, archaic, inefficient, ineffective, and unresponsive system and saw that a total reformulation was necessary. It required a cultural shift, a new way of seeing and doing and believing. He sought transparency at all operational levels, and enlightened leadership that recognized that the system must predominate over the particulars. As he performed his complex task, he formed important rules, and inclusiveness, communication, transparency, and integrity were his pillars, his first principles.

The transformation of Current Medicine requires something similar. Deming's most famous principle, "In God we trust; all others must bring data," must underlie the medical transition. Our current medical model arose not as a result of careful empirical planning, but as a result of expedient reactive actions that did not necessarily serve the greater good. With our recently expanding science base we are newly able to justify the Serenity Prayer's injunction to know the difference between what is changeable and what is not. As we learn what actually determines health, we are at a critical point where we can direct resources to what is possible.

Deming's strategy for transformation insists upon inclusiveness. In the same way, Next Medicine means shared rights and shared responsibilities. Each part of the medical continuum—patient, provider, and community—needs to be examined systematically. If we turned Deming loose on our present situation, he would start by identifying the elements that need to be fixed.

The three separate but unequal components of Next Medicine are the individual, the *sine qua non* of what I call the Commonhealth; the medical profession, defining and assuring the potential of the individual; and society. These are the anatomic parts from which the whole is created. Let's start by examining the individual.

## Next Medicine's Refocus: Self-Efficacy

Twenty-some years ago, I attended a Stanford Department of Medicine conference on rheumatoid arthritis, that awful crippling, disfiguring, painful condition that affects predominantly women. The lecture followed the standard format: "The best medication is X, the best diet is Y, the best physical therapy is Z." But the conclusion was surprising: "More important than all of these key factors," the lecturer said, "is a well-developed sense of self-efficacy." When I heard that last term, "self-efficacy," I sat bolt upright in my seat. I had spent decades deliberating upon and inquiring into the multiple positive and negative features (determinants) of life, but self-efficacy was a new and riveting term for me. Self-efficacy. It sounds like an erudite, vacuous, scholarly term of little relevance. But just a moment's reflection leads to the recognition that self-efficacy is the centerpiece, the keystone on which all other body and mind functions depend. Self-efficacy: self-sufficiency, intactness, wholeness, autonomy, independence. These concepts embody the essence of what it means to be fully alive, fully functional.

I am immensely fortunate to have the noted authority Albert Bandura, emeritus professor at Stanford, close at hand (12). He is the most cited psychologist in the world and has made self-efficacy his life's labor. He has written many dozens of scholarly papers and books on the core elements of human psychological functioning. Self-efficacy, he says, is health. Health is self-efficacy. Rather than being a remote scholarly label, it comes close to being the central axis for health and for Next Medicine.

It is also subject to empirical study. By means of carefully designed questions, Bandura can assign a person an efficacy score. He writes a prescription for self-efficacy just as I write one for penicillin. The four core ingredients are (1) small steps of mastery, (2) peer examples, (3) social persuasion, and (4) diminishment of cues of failure. In other words: first, do not try to run a mile right away; walk to the mailbox and then work up from there. Second, look around you and take cues from others who have built their competence. Third, social persuasion means developing a markedly greater health literacy and personal responsibility to act on the behaviors that determine health, and not delegating health to the medical-industrial complex. Fourth, do not accept a pain in your foot as a reason to stop walking. Get a pair of shoes that fit, walk more slowly—but walk. Taken together, these four principles specify how the most disenfranchised individuals can reach their potential.

When we lose self-efficacy, we cede competence to agencies beyond ourselves. We offload self-care to others. John Gardner recalled a conversation he had with Martin Luther King, Jr. at a conference called, "First, Teach Them to Read." King whispered in Gardner's ear, "First teach them to believe in themselves" (13). Humans are born perfect with very few exceptions and, as John Knowles, past president of the Rockefeller Institute, has said, we are made imperfect by our own actions and inactions (14). We fail to preserve our essential nature. Out of ignorance and laziness we have forfeited our intrinsic gift of healing. We have neglected our nature, that perfection of form and function that has been deeded to us by millions of years of evolutionary challenge, acceptance, and rejection.

Maintaining our individual quota of energy exchange is self-efficacy. A limb in a cast withers quickly, just as our whole body withers when removed from the challenging world. Self-efficacy is the maintenance and extension of our coping competence, which is revealed mostly under challenge. We must reclaim control.

We cannot wait until 70% of our reserve capacity is exhausted to resume self-care. We are fortunate that our renewal capacity is so robust, but deferring or postponing self-care is a hazardous business. Every physician recalls situations when patients presented with what should have been a self-limiting illness, only to find the person overcome by a lesser insult, all fundamentally the result of a failure to assert self-efficacy.

Psychologist Martin Seligman's description of the helpless/hopeless syndrome is not just poetry (15). It is an empirically demonstrable biological state with hard biomarkers. The learned helplessness of today's Disease Medicine patient results from being bombarded by hints of failure, which the media multiply. Suggestions of disease become self-fulfilling.

We are fortunate that we have clear preventive and therapeutic strategies available. Bandura emphatically denies the inevitability of loss, the idea that "you can't change human nature." If helplessness can be learned, it can be unlearned. Self-efficacy is a suit of armor against the welter of assaults on our health competence. The fact that 60% of those who visit a doctor have dominant lifestyle issues (poor diet, physical inactivity, smoking) is a testament to the epidemic nature of low efficacy. Self-efficacy, in and of itself, is a major preventive medicine, both a strong vaccination and a strong therapy. Surgeons can predict the postoperative course of their patients on the basis of the patients' preoperative attitudes and psychological patterns. Bandura's four steps to self-efficacy need to be on every refrigerator door, the first prescription written every time. When I asked him recently when I could stop working on my efficacy, he replied, "Never."

Kate Lorig, a Stanford epidemiologist, has taken self-efficacy to the crucial domain of chronic disease management (16). Chronic illness is a big-ticket item, yet the medical treatments we have for it are poor. Take congestive heart failure. Any young physician can write a 10-page essay on medical management of congestive heart failure, an $80 billion to $200 billion annual enterprise. Yet for all the technical brilliance of our clinical strategies, they are secondary to the actions of the individual who has the condition and is an intimate participant in the therapeutic protocol.

Chronic disease management is Lorig's forte, and she has broken new ground in the field. Numerous small-scale demonstrations of the superiority of enhanced self-efficacy have now led to its large-scale implementation, notably in Great Britain, where the Health Ministry has decreed the Expert Patient protocol, a detailed curriculum of self-help, to be the standard of care.

This example of a behaviorally driven "best practice" applies to virtually every participant in Disease Medicine. Every tenet of Disease Medicine is upgraded when we include self-efficacy within its "scientific" rubric. I would estimate that Lorig's and other's self-management strategies have done more for the good of their patients than all the MDs nearby.

## Next Medicine's Refocus II: Personal Responsibility

Hand in hand with the principle of self-efficacy goes personal responsibility. Several years ago I had the opportunity to appear on CNN's *Sonya Live*, a TV show out of New York. I was perched on a stool in the CNN studio on lower California Street in San Francisco, and Sonya and her audience were connected to me by a TV monitor. My task was to construct a scenario for how all of us can live to be 100, healthy and happy and generally pleased with our lives. My opening statement on the subject lasted maybe 8 or 9 minutes. When I finished, I felt that I had done an adequate job of establishing how we all ought to be able to join in the celebration of my optimistic forecasts. Sonya dutifully thanked me for my remarks and then turned to a young woman who was propped in the front row of the audience and asked her, "What do you think about what Dr. Bortz just said?" With great animation, the woman replied, "I don't believe a word he said. These doctors all think they're so smart, but they don't know what they're talking about. Have you ever met an old doctor? All old doctors are dead." She continued without pause, "Every time I feel like taking a walk, I lie down. And I love fat." Her girth was ample testimony to this fact.

By this time the woman had the whole audience pumped up, having punctured this pompous medical professor from Stanford. Sonya turned back to me and asked me what I had to say about these remarks. I'm sure that I must have been slack-jawed as I searched for a response, any response. I stammered, "Well, first as an American I must respect the right of anyone to say whatever they wish." I scrambled. "But I also believe that with rights come responsibilities, and when you're not responsible, you forfeit the right." What? What did I just say? Dead air, and a hurried station break.

I was alone in the San Francisco studio with this very aggressive statement delivered on nationwide TV still ringing in my ears. Had I spoken badly and been crudely obnoxious in my reaction? Had I offended everybody? When the station break ended, the program continued with a few callow pleasantries to defuse the earlier tension I had created. The program had certainly not anticipated this spontaneous outburst on my part. Nor had I. Yet the longer I reflected on what had happened, the prouder I became of my response. Rights ultimately derive from responsibilities, and when you are not responsible, you forfeit the right. Yes! I have made this axiom my worldview and believe that it is directly relevant to our present medical mess.

A steady stream of medical gurus have agreed that the individual is primarily responsible for his or her own health. In 1977, John Knowles, former president of Rockefeller University and chief of Massachusetts General Hospital, wrote: "The next major event in the health of the American people will come from the assumption of one's own health and the necessary changing of habits for the majority of Americans" (17). Victor Fuchs, senior economist at the Bureau of Economic Research, has asserted that "the largest potential gain in health of the American people will derive from their assumption of responsibility for their lifestyle" (18). And Robert Blank, professor of politics at the University of Canterbury in New Zealand, wrote, "Although people have a right to design their own lifestyle, if they choose to engage in practices and behaviors that put them at higher risk, they should be prepared to relinquish their claim on societal health care resources. By failing to balance their rights with responsibilities, they will surrender positive extension of their rights. The concept of responsibilities places rights in a social context" (19).

The emphatic statements of that *Sonya* audience member may have been all right 20 or 50 years ago, when we really did not know enough to require people to preserve their health. Having such a shallow base of competence placed us all at risk of the whims of fate so that individual rights took precedence. The woman's rejection of any authority to challenge her right to self-abuse was sanctioned in the past. I have had the opportunity to discuss my hang-up regarding the *Sonya* encounter with Harvard bioethicist Norman Daniels, John Rawls's successor in the Harvard social justice tradition (20). I asked him whether it was not time to expect, if not demand, something of Tilly so that she would change her self-destructive lifestyle. Can't society encourage or expect her to live responsibly? Daniels was not at all sympathetic to my query. He thought that my view of her irresponsibility was actually "blaming the victim." To me this was like saying, "Dr. Bortz, how can you expect that woman to be responsible when she and millions like her are so disenfranchised by our culture that her lifestyle of immediate gratification is predictable?"

I spent a lot of time pondering this intersection of rights and responsibilities. It reminded me of an unusual clinical experience I once had. About 30 years ago, when I was on the teaching service at Stanford Medical Center, a 20-year-old man was admitted to our unit from the emergency room. He was suffering from what turned out to be acute bacterial endocarditis (ABE), a virulent infection of the lining and valves of the heart. He had shown up in the emergency room desperately sick with chills and tremors and on the verge of shock. The diagnosis of ABE was quickly established and the care team was mobilized. Critical to his history was that he was an acknowledged intravenous heroin addict. His unsanitary self-injections gave bacteria easy access to his circulatory system. Blood cultures quickly revealed the specific nature of the infecting bug. Unfortunately, our medical endeavors were insufficient to reverse the sepsis, so we consulted the cardiac surgery team, who vigorously scraped the infection from the interior of his heart and replaced the torn valve.

Postoperatively he did well and was released, but within several days he was back. Our patient was re-injecting drugs, even though this was what had led to his earlier problem. In another major operation, surgeons implanted a new heart valve. In a week or so he stabilized enough to go home. Predictably, within a month he was back in the emergency room, again with ABE. A similar surgical rescue was performed. A third heart valve was implanted. After this encounter, the medical residents presented his case at our weekly grand medical rounds—not as a clinical challenge, as we were very aware of the technical requirements of each episode—but as a psychosocial dilemma, asking whether he had the right to continue his self-destructive behavior when this assertion of his personal privilege cost so much in energy and money. He, of course, paid nothing for all his bills, which probably came to about $50,000 per valve. They were assumed by Medicaid—or, in effect, the American taxpayers.

Which medical text or lecture or article could guide us? Did we need a sheriff or a heart surgeon? We felt impotent. Then our patient disappeared; he did not come back to the emergency room. Had he died? Had he moved? One of our enterprising medical residents called the Los Angeles County Hospital and learned that he had taken up his dangerous behavior again. This sorry case history provides volumes of materials for moral and practical speculation on the issue of medical futility. This is a prime topic in any discussion of medical ethics. Must we treat the untreatable? Try to cure the incurable? Certainly our patient was treatable—but at what cost?

A second similar case followed shortly afterward. A severe alcoholic was repeatedly admitted to our unit as we watched his liver gradually disintegrate. Once again, his personality was exuberant and his intellectual brilliance made his case more challenging. I made the mistake of becoming personally involved in his well-being and arranged for a consultation in the liver transplant facility at the University of California San Francisco. It was his one opportunity for life. On his way to the consult he stopped at a bar and got drunk, effectively nullifying his chances for a second chance.

Extending these cases to my TV show adversary on the *Sonya* set is a big stretch. But in the abstract, her behavior will cost her and the rest of us extravagantly in the years ahead. Taken to the extreme, self-abuse can preoccupy society's energies and resources to such an extent that there will not be enough left over for it to sustain itself.

Recently, in their *New England Journal of Medicine* article, Emanuel and Fuchs provocatively asked, "Who is really paying the medical bills?" (21). All of us are paying the bills in one guise or another. Daily our local news stations

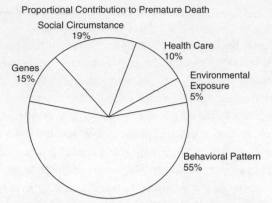

Proportional Contribution to Premature Death

**Figure 6.1** Contribution to premature death. From "We Can Do Better—Improving the Health of the American People," *New England Journal of Medicine*, September 2007, Volume 357, page 1222. Copyright © 2007, Massachusetts Medical Society. All rights reserved.

report on how public school teachers are suffering from cutbacks in funds. In a report for the Health Improvement Institute, medical statesman Donald Berwick relates how Massachusetts, with its generally acclaimed universal health coverage plan, is now running a $2 billion deficit, which is imperiling the state subsidy for heating oil for the poor. This is an unexpected, but real, negative tradeoff.

In 1977, John Knowles (17) wrote, "The cost of individual irresponsibility for health has become prohibitive. The choice is individual responsibility or social failure." Responsibility and duty must be given parity with rights and freedom. I contend that the moment is now. We must look at reality and set boundaries on an individual's right to self-abuse in order to bring the spiraling social costs of harmful behaviors under control. We might reduce the message to, "If you want to kill yourself, go ahead, but don't send me or anybody else your bill." My view is that the rights/responsibility debate can no longer be filibustered. *Laissez-faire* has consequences. We all laud America's unique heritage of personal rights and individual freedoms. Patrick Henry was a great hero, but even he might defer to the more encompassing mandate of personal responsibility. Responsibility derives directly from knowledge. Benjamin Franklin asked how a newborn can be held responsible for anything. But as we age, life's curriculum demands responsibility.

Much has been made of the idea of "nature's lottery," the seemingly capricious nature of illness. But defaulting to such fatalism masks the reality of our new ability to choose health, a choice made possible by the fact that we know the details of health—its origins, its language, and its metrics. It is a choice that is central to Next Medicine.

As the core principles of the science of biology were being revealed, an unexpected radical realization came to light once again. Aristotle had warned that we cannot understand an object simply by breaking it down into its parts, that we must also analyze it as a whole (1). But we had lost sight of this admonition over time: it had been progressively obscured by the startling new features that our scientific tools, especially the microscope and the telescope, revealed. As our eyes have grown accustomed to the new depths of field these magnifications have opened up, our memory of the whole has been diminished. Unquestionably, the reductionism habit paid off, with huge intellectual gains. Turning up the power of our instrumentation made profound insight possible. But taking apart a body's hundred trillion cells, or the universe electron by electron, followed by further dissection to even smaller components, does not explain how a body or the universe works. As Einstein said, "Not everything that counts can be counted, and not everything that can be counted counts" (2). We cannot understand an electric motor or an elephant by analyzing only its parts.

In his famous 1972 *Science* article "More Is Different," Philip Anderson recognized the importance of the concept of "emergence" (3). This is the reverse of reductionism. In his book *The Emergence of Everything*, Harold Morowitz details 28 separate levels of nature's process, framed in an almost linear chronological sequence from the beginning of the universe to the level we now occupy, from atomic grouping to the search for spirit, or something in that domain (4).

Within this analysis the human phylogenetic line has many emergent steps—from lemur to Lucy to us. The inevitable questions: after us, *Homo sapiens*, what is the next emergent level? How does simplicity generate complexity? How does chemistry generate biology? Atoms generate molecules that generate elements that generate compounds that generate cells and tissues that generate organs that generate organisms. In evolution, fish yielded amphibians, which yielded reptiles, which yielded birds and mammals and us, each new entity containing its additionally complex organizing principles, rules yielding what has been called "the combinatorial explosive" essence of life. Even Pope John Paul II acknowledged the significance of emergence in his encyclical *Fides et Ratio* in 1998 (5).

Richard Dawkins makes the point that memes, the culturally generated items of inheritance, tools, and behavioral novelty markedly speed up emergence (6). These punctuations of equilibrium often generate unexpected and unpredictable consequences, both bad and good. The term "co-evolution" captures how emergence is the result of the complex interrelationships between organisms and the environment, between nature and nurture (7).

But the crux is that whereas each of the individual steps is separate, analysis does not extrapolate to the layers immediately above or below. In as much as life is one of the intermediary foci of Morowitz's scheme, I embrace the concept of life as an emergent phenomenon, not predictable or identifiable by surveys of domains above and below, and thereby requiring its own explanatory system. This certainly does not claim that adjacent levels of explication are not helpful, but they must be integrated into a definition of life as a whole.

As energy passes through different levels of matter, it changes. In her book *The Rainbow and the Worm*, Mae Wan Ho, director of the Bioelectrodynamics Laboratory at the Open University in Britain, repeatedly characterizes matter as stored energy (8)—so as new forms of matter change, energy emerges in different distributions. The ascending and descending hierarchical levels are distinct, but they are also interdependent. There are connections between the levels and the separate parts. And so we come to the second major concept (after emergence) underpinning Next Medicine: thermodynamics.

## The Thermodynamics of Next Medicine: Energy and Life

In February 1943, Erwin Schrodinger, a displaced Austrian physicist whose pioneering theories provided the foundation for much of contemporary quantum physics, delivered a series of lectures at Trinity College in Dublin entitled, "What Is Life? The Physical Aspects of the Living Cell" (9). While acknowledging the poverty of classical physics in providing a working format for life, he incorporated thermodynamics into the operating manual for living systems. Building on the thermodynamic work of Boltzman, Gibbs, and Maxwell, who had discovered the physical laws underlying the behavior of heat and energy, Schrodinger extended their concepts, which were largely derived from analyzing mechanical systems such as steam engines. The energy flows of an engine, however, represent an isolated state and are therefore only partially comparable to living systems.

Schrodinger's subsequent, now legendary book *What Is Life?* broke the conceptual logjam. It provided an emergent level of understanding of life, health, and all the rest of the natural world. The second law of thermodynamics as applied to the process of living provides a new and rich explanatory platform. Schrodinger's book brought us to the necessary emergent hierarchical level for discussing life, health, birth, death, and aging in an entirely scientific context. Within the parameters of the Second Law of Thermodynamics reside the necessary fundamentals that allow a coherent understanding of basic matters that have preoccupied humankind from our earliest beginnings. British physicist and author C. P. Snow once remarked, "A person who is not familiar with the laws of thermodynamics is equivalent to a person who has never read Shakespeare" (10).

Classical thermodynamics deals largely with systems in equilibrium. Life clearly is not a state of equilibrium. Similarly, thermodynamics was first invoked to understand closed systems that have no exchange with the environment—which again is only limitedly comparable to living systems. Yet Schrodinger incorporated energy, matter, time, and space into a formulaic effort to define life. That these are the basic fundamental variables in solving life's equation is a key concept, but we need to further refine the appropriate hierarchical level.

Ilya Prigogine, winner of the 1977 Nobel Prize in chemistry, sought to integrate these components into his redefinition of the Second Law (11). He, like Newton, had to create a new vocabulary for his views. *Dissipative structures*, *bifurcation points*, and *order through fluctuation* are all terms he invented to describe how the features of energy are grafted onto life processes. But Prigogine's upgrading of Schrodinger is insufficient. Mae Wan Ho (8), Jeffrey Wicken (12), Peter Corning (13), and Harold Morowitz (4), those excellent explicators of nature's designs, offer a new emphasis on energy flow, not simply on energy as an entity, but as a dynamic unidirectional component. Further, matter should not be defined as a closed unchanging feature but must be considered as a continuum with energy. Mae Wan Ho, as I have said, considers matter to be stored energy. Matter is available energy. Energy is the ability to do work. Matter and energy both flow.

If we take this seemingly esoteric science to the operational level, we can define life as an emergent property of an organism that functions between certain set boundaries. Morowitz writes extensively about "pruning" parameters, by which he illustrates that the flow of energy and matter over time is not free to pursue random paths and combinations, but is constrained by physical laws, gravity, and other physical rules, which reign in most theoretical chemical processes.

A crucial modifying consideration of the "life as self-organization theme" is that life is directed by deterministic laws. Schrodinger amazingly guessed this critical fact by proposing "aperiodic crystals" as the agents that specify life. They set limited parameters. This was more elegantly discerned in the elaboration of the famous double helix of DNA, and RNA. These key molecules contain the structuring rules of what is possible. The genes make and enforce structural and operational rules, but they themselves are byproducts of such rules, the networks of life that of themselves mean little. Only when genes are inserted into a grand operatic operational ensemble do they achieve the acclaim that their ardent supporters have extravagantly claimed for them.

Five years ago I had a unique opportunity to talk with the physicist and mathematician Freeman Dyson for an hour as we sat together on the runners' bus awaiting the start of the Boston Marathon in Hopkinton. Dyson, whom Nobel physicist Steven Weinberg called "the best living physicist never to have won a Nobel Prize" (15), was there attending his wife Ibby, who is a distinguished senior female marathon competitor. She and I were to approach the starting line in an hour or so. In the meantime, I had the very special chance to scan Dyson's particular version of genesis, entitled *Origins of Life*, which he published in 1985 (16). In it he juxtaposes the two central players in the origin of life, metabolism (chemistry) and replication (physiology). "The history of life is counterpoint music, a two-part invention with two voices," he writes. In this, Dyson borrowed from the mathematician John von Neumann's response to the question of life's origin: "Life is not one thing but two," metabolism and replication, distinct and separate (17). This raises the question: which came first, the chicken or the egg?

Dyson comes down on the side of metabolism being first. Shortly after Schrodinger's 1943 lectures, von Neumann postulated an analogy between living organisms and a mechanical automaton. As in von Neumann's automatons, the computer industry has adapted two components: hardware and software. This is exactly analogous to living cells, whose hardware is proteins, and software nucleotides. Dyson conjectured that chemical Genesis occurred rapidly and probably more than once. The precise earliest moment when life-sustaining metabolism was hatched is obscure, but probably it arose in a deep hot hole in the ocean floor. The most ancient lineage of bacteria are thermo-philes that are specialized to grow in hot environments close to the boiling point of water. Dyson acknowledges the speculative nature of this musing, but it is certainly alien to our bucolic Garden of Eden obstetrical suite. He further conjectured that the first replicating system was composed of a few hundred molecules that, by scavenging and coalescing, transduced themselves into something resembling a living cell.

Dyson recalls Darwin's answer to the "what is life?" question as that "tangled bank of grasses and flowers and bees and butterflies growing in profusion with-out any discernible pattern achieving homeostasis by means of a web of inter-dependency (synergy) too complicated for us to unravel" (18). Freeman's creation account is a modern synthesis of function and reproduction, the origins of life, how we work and how we pass on our energies to subsequent versions of ourselves.

Similarly, in 2002, Dan Koshland, a molecular biologist at the University of California Berkeley, published a perspective of the definition of life in *Science*, where he had served as editor (19). Koshland wrote that "a living organism is an organized unit which carries out metabolic reactions, defends itself against injury, responds to stimuli, and has the capacity to be at least a partner in repro-duction." He labels the essential principles as thermodynamic and kinetic (note the energetic emphasis). Koshland is dissatisfied with his own reductionist effort, and elaborates, "Life has seven pillars: program, improvisation, compart-mentalization, energy, regeneration, adaptability, and seclusion, the fundamental principles on which a living system is based" (19).

Since I have covered energy, in what follows I will focus on certain aspects of improvisation, compartmentalization, regeneration, and adaptability as they relate to human health. Our redesigned support structures are homeodynamics, plasticity, and symmorphosis.

## Stable Change: Homeodynamics

One of the problems in the study of nature is that it does not seem to stand still while we measure it. Time's arrow never hangs idle. Nature is always on the move. For instance, the basic biochemical machine of life, the Krebs cycle, turns over 2,000 times a second (20), 12,000 rpm. Empirically, we seek understand-ing by reducing nature's complexity to the simplest, most stable model. And surely nature provides marvelous evidence of stability. The 19th-century scien-tist Claude Bernard, considered the father of physiology, is famous for his description of the constancy of the internal milieu, its *fixité* (21). His focus was on the organism's ability to remain upright while being buffeted by wide-ranging environmental challenges. His work led to Walter Cannon's celebration of this capacity, codified in 1921 as homeostasis, the body's ability to maintain its function at altitude, temperature extremes, nutritional stress, and the like, ever ready in the effort to sustain itself in the face of daunting external challenge (22).

This concept was incorporated into medical lore. I was taught homeostasis in my second-year medical school physiology class. What we were taught was crude, and has been critically updated by F. Eugene Yates, a physiologist and professor of medicine at UCLA (23). I first learned of Yates when he wrote an accompanying editorial to an article I had written for the *Journal of the American Geriatrics Society*, "The Physics of Frailty," in 1993 (24). After immediately contacting Yates, I was introduced to his formulation of homeodynamics, which I initially grasped as a replacement for the scientifically incorrect term of homeostasis. Simply stated, there is no stasis in life. It is alien to all things in the universe, particularly life. Life is anything but static—it is defined by flux, by thresholds and gradients, and not by set, fixed points.

Yates's wonderful term "homeodynamics" expanded the description of the stabilizing property of life a thousand-fold. Stability is not an emergent property of inertia, but rather of the entire interrelated hierarchy of natural processes. Homeodynamics describes how the organism is at once both plastic and reactive, stable and functional. Homeodynamics explains how matter and energy truly interact, and is thus a richer term than homeostasis. Yates's efforts have done much to illumine my primary field of geriatrics as his reach to the processes of aging, senescence, frailty, and eventually death provides a rigorous platform for empirical exploration.

In their progressive elaboration of homeodynamics, Bernard, Cannon, and Yates insist that the organism is the reference structure, not its components— how the whole works as a functional unity, matter and energy interacting within a complex feedback structure.

One of these crucial feedback structures is our use of oxygen, an example of homeodynamics. In *The Origins of Human Disease*, Thomas McKeown, a professor of social medicine at the University of Birmingham in England, observes that an animal has four central needs: oxygen, food, water, and warmth (25). Of these, oxygen is a given; the other three needs all require directed adaptive behaviors, including migration. But regardless of where a creature lives, except below water or above 11,000 feet in altitude, it has a sufficient supply of oxygen. This omnipresence translates into the organism's small reserve capacity. An organism's survival capacity when deprived of any of the four needs is inversely related to its general availability. Food, water, and temperature demand some adaptive capacity. Oxygen does not, and consequently animals have no reserve tank of it and succumb within 4 minutes if deprived of it, like a candle under a jelly glass. An organism's ability to maintain its vital supply of oxygen involves a complex multi-step process, beginning with the respiratory tubes, circulatory equipment, blood cell membranes, and finally the intracellular machinery, which extracts oxygen from its hemoglobin carriage, which then sparks the familiar equation of life. Sugar plus oxygen yields carbon dioxide and water and adenosine triphosphate (ATP). This high-school chemistry is the general process by which we live. It cannot proceed adequately without oxygen.

## Plasticity

The central concept of homeodynamics leads directly to the important topic of phenotypic plasticity, the capacity of all organisms to adapt to their environments (26). This core principle encapsulates the adaptability of all natural processes and is central to the definition of life. All living creatures exhibit plasticity. The plasticity of plants is extensively studied as seeds of a particular species exhibit extraordinary developmental variance when grown in different environments. Levels of messenger RNA rise 150-fold within 20 minutes of mechanical stimulation of the leaves or stem of *Arabidopsis*, a flowering plant of the mustard family (27). Over the decades, studies at the Carnegie laboratories at Stanford have shown how the simple seeds of the mustard plant exhibit profound morphologic differences depending on whether they are grown at sea level or in the foothills of the Sierra Nevada.

Animals have the additional adaptive capacity of movement to accommodate to their environments. Migrating birds, hibernating bears, and snakes show marked seasonal variability in their nutritional habitats. UCLA's Jared Diamond studied the python; within 1 to 2 days of consuming an entire yearly food ration in a single gulp, it shows a doubling of its small intestinal mass, a 6-fold increase in microvillous length, a 5- to 40-fold increase in glucose and amino acid transporters of the mucosa, and an increase of oxygen consumption that is 44 times the basal level (28). Studies of the digestive organ mass in the red knot, a long-distance migrating shorebird, show predictable structural changes in the pre-and post-flight periods. Experimental resection of portions of the small intestine in rats leads to virtually total restitution of absorptive capacity within 1 week. Extreme structural and functional reactivity to fuel load, therefore, is impressively demonstrable across a broad spectrum of life forms.

Skeletogenesis is the best-studied model of animal phenotypic plasticity. In 1876, the German physician and anatomist Julius Wolff proposed the law that still bears his name: "The robustness of any bone is in direct proportion to the physical forces which affect it" (29). Computer simulations of embryonic bone development at the Stanford School of Engineering have determined that the eventual construct conforms precisely to the vector forces applied to the bone during development (30). Similarly, studies of bone development at cellular and subcellular levels reveal that the intracellular anatomy of interconnected micro-filaments and microtubules, the cytoskeleton, is in direct proportion to the forces applied by a process that Buckminster Fuller termed "tensegrity" in his work on force and form (31).

Such forces act to push and pull cells in their matrix into relative positions that facilitate chemical gradients and physical patterns. These gradients involve growth factors, cytokines, and circulatory and metabolic adaptations. Receptors transform energy into a form that facilitates biological receptivity, which is generally chemical in nature. The repackaged energy acts to turn on the nuclear gene expression machinery, leading to structural reactivity and cellular growth. Structure thereby reflects need. Figure 7.1 illustrates how the organism captures various environmental stimuli and translates them directly into appropriate conforming structure.

This far-reaching reconceptualization describes how spatiotemporal organization evolves out of the interreactions between matter and energy. Structure is dynamic and becomes stable through its activity. Supramolecular organization derives from an energy flow on individual atoms and molecules. This ordering effect of an energy flow on matter seems counterintuitive, but it remains one of the more profound observations ever made. All of life is essentially made from the same small set of molecules, the same starting material. The variety of life therefore derives not so much from different building blocks but from how the environment serves to shape the basic matter. This is phenotypic plasticity.

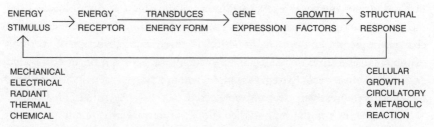

Conversion of Energetic Stimulus to Structure

**Figure 7.1** Phenotypic plasticity. From "The Physics of Frailty," *Journal of the American Geriatrics Society*, September 1993, Volume 41, page 1006.

How does the environment affect structure? The molecular biology of this shaping action is just emerging. We know that every cell in nature is affected by energy forces, some, like those associated with the musculoskeletal system, more obviously than others. But even the mucosal cells of the gastrointestinal tract are regularly exposed to the push and pull of peristaltic activity, as well as the endothelial cells of the vascular system and changes in blood flow.

This last statement underlines an important experiment that was conducted here at Stanford. Fifty years ago, I was struck by an article in the *New England Journal of Medicine* about "Mr. Marathon" (32). It was written by Dr. Paul Dudley White, the doctor who treated Eisenhower after his heart attack in 1953, and his colleagues. The article presented the autopsy findings on Clarence DeMar, a legendary hero to all of us who have run the Boston Marathon. He ran it 32 times and won it 7 times. He was famous throughout the running community. He died at age 70 of colon cancer in 1958. His autopsy showed nothing remarkable except for the size of his arteries, which were abnormally large. White's article featured pictures of DeMar's coronary arteries and proposed that his prodigious running had literally reshaped them. This modest single case report got hardly a ripple of reaction in the medical world, but it was of such interest to me that I tore it out almost as a curiosity.

I started to run when I was 40 as a form of grief sublimation after my father died. I was aware that exercise was a non-traditional, non-pharmaceutical home treatment for depression. So, being a Walter Mitty pseudo-athlete, I set my cap to run the Boston Marathon that year, 1971. It was so rewarding that I have sustained the habit and have run a marathon a year for the past 40 years. More impressively, my petite wife has caught the bug and has also immersed herself in the running world. Our approach is different. She wants to win; I want to finish. But her winning urge has resulted in two wins in Boston for the over-60 and subsequently over-70 female. So I sleep every night with a double winner of the Boston Marathon, which is intimidating. Further, it is our claim to fame that we are the only married couple over 70 ever to have completed this fabled run, a feat celebrated in the centerfold of *Runner's World* magazine in 2004.

Ruth Anne's exploits have gone beyond marathons, however, and have extended to participation in the famous Western States Endurance Run through the Sierras, starting at Squaw Valley and ending 100 miles later in Auburn, California. This event has become part of a yearly tradition for us as first our son completed it, leading to my wife's entry and double finishes. The other runners in this heroic undertaking have become our friends.

My encounter with the DeMar article took on new significance. The idea that exercise might change the configuration of the coronary arteries had lain fallow for 40 years. But science had provided exciting new tools to push this observation to the next step. Ed Alderman, head of the cardiac catheterization laboratory at Stanford, had developed a technique to quantify the cross-sectional area of the coronary artery at catheterization time. I proposed to him that I gather up some of our 100-mile runners and do coronary artery visualizations to see whether they confirmed the observation on DeMar.

Twelve of our runner fraternity eagerly volunteered, and before I knew it we were under way. I was at the cath table when Alderman shot the dye into the root of the arteries of our first guinea pig. Poof! There was a sudden and uncharacteristic gush visible on the fluoroscope. I was alarmed: had we inadvertently killed this unwitting subject? But the gush was merely the first evidence of the large blood vessels he presented, as did the others. We published the results of this study in the medical journal *Circulation* in 1993 in an article entitled "Coronary Artery Size and Dilating Capacity in Ultradistance Runners" (33). We had confirmed and extended the 50-year-old findings on DeMar.

What we saw in our study was an outstanding example of phenotypic plasticity. In this case it was the artery size that represented the structural response to an environmental challenge. The challenge was the increased blood flow to the arteries initiated by the exercise load. The endothelial lining cells of the interior of the artery contain receptor sites. These sense their environment just as do those of every cell, plant, and animal. The environment of the inside of an artery is blood flow, so as the blood flow increases, the receptor sites sense this and signal the energy flow to the DNA of the artery wall, which reshapes the artery to accommodate the increased need. Our demonstration has been upgraded by the dissection of the molecular details of the enlarging field of vascular remodeling. We now know, in minute detail, the molecular mechanisms responsible for such an accommodative process.

Another fascinating example of phenotypic plasticity concerns the brain. For a long time, I have had a deep interest in how the brain responds to its environment. I was aware early of the work of Dr. Marian Diamond of the University of California Berkeley. I found her seminal work on the effect of enrichment and deprivation on the brain structure of rats immensely interesting. Her experiments consisted of simply putting rats in different environments, one enriched and the other deprived (34). What is an enriched rat? It is one with cage-mates, toys, and an exercise wheel. What is a deprived rat? It is one in isolation, with no stimuli. Rats from each group were put to a standard maze test. The enriched rats blazed their way through the maze as though they had a MapQuest routing in front of them. The deprived rats bumped their way through the maze and eventually got to the far end by default. The conclusion: enrichment makes you smarter, if you are a rat. Diamond then autopsied the rats and found that the enriched rats had greater brain weight. And when she examined the brain cells under a microscope, she found that the dendritic branchings were exuberant, much like a shrub in springtime; the deprived rats' brain cells looked like stunted twigs. Diamond has expanded her findings and published them in her book, *Magic Trees of the Mind,* in which she elaborates on this plasticity of the stimulated brain (35).

The implications of this are broad. The piano student learns by practice. Professional violinists' brains show structural alterations in the part involved with the busy left hand. Diamond had the opportunity to examine parts of Einstein's brain; whereas the brain *in toto* seemed unremarkable, the parts particularly involved with computational functions were physically enlarged (36).

There are other examples. Consider the story of Kim Peek, portrayed by Dustin Hoffman in the movie *Rain Man*. Kim, whose death from a heart attack at age 58 was covered by the *New York Times*, was born with major brain damage, specifically to the part of the brain that connects the two halves. This defect led to lifelong motor difficulty, resulting in problems in walking and dressing himself. In psychological testing he scored below average on general IQ tests. However, he had a prodigious memory capability, "the Everest of Memory." From the age of 16 months he had a remarkable capacity for memorizing things. He read a book in an hour and remembered 98% of what he read, having memorized vast amounts of information on wide-ranging topics. He could recall 12,000 books from memory. Although not a musical prodigy, he started to play the piano and remembered music that he heard decades ago and could play to the extent permitted by his limited physical dexterity.

Peek underwent neuroimaging of his brain to define the specific pathways of loss and gain. His savant syndrome, sometimes termed "islands of genius," was under continuing scientific study. It occurs much more frequently in males and is related to autism. It occurs in 1 of every 2,000 persons with mental retardation (37).

I have been similarly stimulated by the book *Wolf Children and Feral Man*, by the Rev. J. A. L. Singh and Prof. Robert Zingg (38). The book tells the story of two children who had been living in the jungles of northern India for an uncertain period of time. These rare tales crop up in our lore back to Romulus and Remus, the wolf children memorialized in Roman legend. In 1920 missionaries were startled when five wolves were followed from their den by two ghostlike creatures with bright, piercing eyes, running on all fours and grunting, who were identified as human. They were both girls, the older being approximately 8 years old, and the younger a year and a half. The mother wolf was so protective that she had to be killed before the missionaries were able to retrieve the children, who shrank from them and screamed.

They came to live with the missionary family, and the book is mostly the narrative of their early days. Returned to civilization, they howled at night and lapped their food. They crawled and were covered with sores. They slept with bent legs and huddled together. They cowered when approached by their care-givers and were easily terrified. After a year, the younger girl died, probably from intestinal worms. Her sister refused to eat and drink and wanted to remain with her dead sibling. But after a few days, the older girl took more kindly to the female missionary. The remainder of the story tells of her slow and mostly inef-fective steps to regain humanity. Nine years later, she too died. No clinical details are provided.

These two extraordinary cases, the savant syndrome and feral children, are recorded here merely as evidence of the extreme plasticity of the human being when confronted with extraordinary circumstances. Every cell in all of nature has on its surface many protein molecules called receptor cells. These cells are spatially and chemically configured in such a way as to serve as transmitters of a particular form of energy. Our retinas have thousands of receptor sites whose job it is to collect the photons of light, direct or reflected, and transform these photons into a usable form of chemical energy that can be conducted over our optic nerves to the occipital lobe of the brain, where we experience vision. Similarly, the nose, the tongue, and the eardrums have appropriate receptor site molecules, which generate our sense system awareness. These receptor sites reflect the organism's window onto the world.

I often choose the Lone Cypress on the 17-Mile Drive in Carmel, California, as a prime example of the crucial signaling provided by receptor sites. The Lone Cypress sits dramatically on its rocky knoll, just south of Carmel Bay. Its sinu-ous yet stately figure adorns countless calendars and travel posters. It leans sternly to the east. The reason for this direction is the receptor sites on the trunk and the branches. These molecules sense their environment, which is domi-nated by the westerly winds coming in off the Pacific Ocean. The Cypress' receptor sites capture this mechanical energy and transmit it to the genetic machinery of the tree, incorporating the data into its structural elements, which cause it to list to the left.

All plants react to where they live, since they lack the reactive repertoire of animals, which move in response to environmental cueing. Plants make do with what they have, building structure *in situ* to maximize their adaptivity. The rain forest, the shrubs, and the weeds in the garden all exploit their receptor sites to glorious effect. The plant world confluence of energy and matter is pretty straightforward. The complexity of the animal world involves a more elaborate reactive format, but it nevertheless follows the rules of nature, conforming to and incorporating energetic stimuli.

## Symmorphosis: Structure Matches Function

I first learned of the term "symmorphosis" when I invited Jared Diamond to Stanford to lecture on his book *Guns, Germs, and Steel*. In the course of researching his background, I found his name on a paper that he had written about this concept, which I now embrace as a unifying concept explaining the energy/ matter interface (39).

Symmorphosis was first described by Ewald Weibel, professor of physiology at the University of Bern, and the esteemed physical anthropologist Dick Taylor of Harvard (40). It states that all components in a linked functional system react in quantitative symmetry with one another when faced with a changing environment. Put simply, structure matches function. Weibel and Taylor conducted experiments that validated the idea that when a particular function—oxygen or fuel use—is altered, all the structural components and related functions involved in the sequence are adjusted via phenotypic plasticity to the new demands. Every complementary function is quantitatively linked for oxygen or food delivery. This means that the respiratory dynamic, the heart action, the arteries, arterioles, membrane thickness, capillary density, intracellular components, all rise and fall together, like the proverbial rowboat in the proverbial tide. Fuel use, however, has an additional step, a storage stage. Additional experiments were needed for this calculation, but when they are incorporated, the basic idea of symmorphosis is confirmed. To recapitulate, a body faced with a constantly changing environment must react precisely and equivalently through mechanisms now described at the molecular level. We are what we do.

At a Harvard Medical School lecture a few years ago, I was adamantly proselytizing the "use it or lose it" mandate. A member of the audience raised her hand and asked, "If who you are is what you do, is it then also true that if you don't, you aren't?" I was grateful for such a marvelous rendering of the energy/ matter interface. Is the face that confronts you in the mirror each morning the same face as yesterday's or tomorrow's? We presume our constancy, but the facts speak otherwise.

As Heraclitus reminds us, you cannot step twice in the same river, "for other waters are ever flowing onto you" (41). It is predicated that 98% of our CHNOPS, our carbon, hydrogen, nitrogen, oxygen and sulfur atoms, are different this year from last year. You are therefore today's edition of you, not last July Fourth's or next Christmas's, but today's explicitly.

A July 2005 paper in *Cell*, from the Karolinska Institute and the Lawrence Livermore Laboratory, uses a unique technique to date a person's cells' birthdays. Nuclear weapons testing in the mid-1950s and early 1960s released large quantities of radioactive carbon into the atmosphere, which was eventually distributed evenly into the atmosphere and hence into us (42). Since the test ban treaty of 1963, there has been negligible further contamination of C-14. The authors of this article used accelerator mass spectrometry to increase the sensitivity of cell-birth dating. Their data suggest that the average age of muscle cells is 15 years; the liver replaces itself every 2 months and the intestinal mucosa every 5 days (cells of tissues exposed directly to the environment are short-lived). Even your skeleton, seemingly your most permanent structure, replaces itself every 6 years. Different parts of the brain turn over at low rates; some showed little or no post-birth replacement. We lose about 1 million cells per second. The body makes 50 g of protein each day. That's enough for a lot of cells. It also gets rid of 50 g of protein per day. That's a lot of cells.

Such cell turnover rates emphasize again that life is a dynamic process intimately mixing matter and energy. As Dorion Sagan says, "The body is not a stable entity but a metastable vortex, a whirlpool of flesh, blood, and bone, mucus, sweat and tears, an agglomeration of ever-changing atoms and cells whose continuous turnover is required to create the appearances of stability" (43).

It really is very smart of nature to make all creatures so homeodynamic, plastic, and symmorphotic. Instead of entrusting the lifelong integrity of all cells to a predestined structural and functional format encoded in our genes, nature provides life with a magnificent ability to adjust to constant and sometimes hostile changes in the environment. It is asking too much of our meager set of 21,000 genes to be clever enough to interpret every signal to every cell with the precision that our three related processes ensure.

Although the plasticity of the human body has received minor interest in the realms of health and medicine (it gets no respect, as it is largely unseen), by its very essence it lays claim to being at the root of the free will/determinism debate. If we were in fact fully fixed and immutable by nature, with nurture having little impact on our codified selves, then life would be much simpler: it would already have been decided for us; life would be a no-option affair.

The variegated pageantry of life gives vivid testimony to all the options in life. Homeodynamics, phenotypic plasticity, and symmorphosis are the expressions of these series of choices. This avalanche of new self-knowledge allows us to shape our lives by choice. We are clearly no longer determined by Fate, and this reality is gathering momentum as we learn more. Choice is highly to be desired, if we know the odds, but we need to be aware of the consequences.

To start a Kuhnian revolution—to overthrow the Current Medicine paradigm in favor of the Next Medicine paradigm—we need to apply this science to clearly defining health. What, after all, is health?

# Unweaving Health | 8

Dr. George Sheehan, guru to a generation of dedicated runners, was a close friend of mine. A cardiologist from Red Bank, New Jersey, Sheehan forsook his medical career at age 60 to preach the gospel of fitness. His Jesuit training provided elegant material for his regular columns in *Runner's World* magazine, as well as his influential book, *Running and Being* (1). Sheehan's life philosophy coincided closely with mine, except for the fact that he was a competitive runner, a heritage from his high-school track team days. I, on the other hand, am glacially slow, fortunate to finish a race before dark. For Sheehan, winning mattered; for me, finishing was the whole game. This different approach to running provided a platform for my advice to him as he was dying slowly from prostate cancer. He became depressed and fatalistic. I urged him to keep going: accept the diagnosis, but reject the verdict.

Fortunately, he listened. Doctors are notoriously terrible patients, but Sheehan managed to maximize the good life before he died. Shortly before that, he related this retrospective summary of his life (2). "Until I was six, life was perfect, Mummy and Daddy were wonderful. My puppy was great fun. My bed was dry. I loved desserts, everything was perfect. But then I turned six, and since then, nothing has been the same. I've pondered long what it was that happened when I turned six, and I finally figured it out. When I was five, all I kept wondering about was 'why.' Why Mommy? Why Daddy? Why everybody?

And then I turned six, and I started to ask how Mommy? How Daddy? How everybody? Instead of chasing answers to the basic big questions of my life, I began to try to figure out all the many daily little problems. Life has never been the same since."

This change in life's basic question, from *why* to *how*, is the source of much of our Current Medicine malaise. In making proximate demands, we forget the ultimate issues. Sheehan's observation is kindred to Nietzsche's assertion that "a person who has a why in life can put up with any how." In approaching the symptoms of Current Medicine, we are stuck on addressing the *how* questions. They provide the wrong keys to the *why* treasure. We need to establish the *why* of the human potential, and the *why* of the human potential is health.

Current Medicine has a consuming insistence on what is wrong, and its principal mission is to seek cures. It is fixated on the acute challenges of daily life, and thereby neglects the attenuated effects of processes that act incrementally over a lifespan. It is derived from a reductionist methodology that emphasizes parts, our components. It is excessively specialized. It fixates on moments, rather than on a whole process. Finally, the locus of control in Current Medicine lies outside, not with, the individual: someone else is in charge of your potential.

Next Medicine mandates a systems approach, insisting on the study of the whole. Next Medicine insists that you are in ultimate control. Control lies within, not outside, the individual.

But merely stating the differences between Current and Next Medicine is not enough. We must apply sturdy science, the science of Health, to support the differing assumptions. Merely adjusting or polishing the precepts of Current Medicine will not sustain a new paradigm. Entirely new definitions are required; new language and new metrics apply.

## A Working Definition of Health

Health, like life, defies a trivial definition. It seems too intimate, too self-evident, too automatic to lend itself to a simple description. In their book *What Is Life?* Lynn Margulis and Dorion Sagan point out that the question itself is a linguistic trap, which seems to demand a noun for a response (3). Yet health, like life, is better described as a verb rather than a noun.

A general search in various reference works for proposed answers to "what is health?" often includes the seemingly perverse advice, "See *sickness*." Yet most people now reject the idea that health is merely the opposite of disease. The World Health Organization offers up instead, "Total well-being, a positive state rather than the absence of a negative state" (4). The Ottawa Charter for Health Promotion of a few years ago echoes the same inclusive definition of health, although it has never gained much traction (5).

Albert Szent Gyorgy, the discoverer of vitamin C, concluded that "Health, to us, is as water is to a fish" (6). Other descriptions include "the gestalt of life," "the highest value," "universal sympathy," Hippocrates' "balance," the Greek "golden mean," "wholeness," and "concealed harmony" (7). Kant, in his *Critique of Pure Reason,* called health "the inner natural perfection" and "the unified organic" (8). Abraham Maslow's "self-actualization" is an appropriate synonym (9). Albert Schweitzer called health "the doctor within" (10). The German philosopher Hans-Georg Gadamer called upon medicine to enhance and embrace this concept, asserting that medicine's highest goal is to surrender control of health to the individual (11). Illich powerfully argued that health belongs to the individual (12).

"A durable capital asset" and "a good investment" describe health in economic terms, and there is utility in this approach, as we will see later. Many define health in more operational terms. René Dubos called health "the ability to function in a manner acceptable to oneself" (13). Such a utilitarian emphasis is that "health is that which works." "The capacity to do work," "efficacy," all are in accord with the suggestion that health is a verb instead of a noun. It is more operational than structural. Defining health in active terms is reflected in Dubos's insistence that health is not a given (fate), but that it must be earned over and over (choice), something that demands action.

More contemporary and scientific definitions of health call it "an emergent dynamic property of the whole organism" (14), "a subtle emergent property of dynamic complexity" (15), "a dynamic coherence" (16), all descriptions that include frontier scientific terminology. Health is "kinetic," otherwise called "an interlocking of interacting nonlinear oscillations" (17), "the generation of global patterns from interacting lower-level composites" (18). Applying the science of the previous chapter, we can define health as "an emergent state of the whole which generates, stabilizes, and maintains the functional potential of the organism through homeodynamically integrated metabolic networks, constrained by genetic rules, and driven by a modulated flow of energy." That is a mouthful, but a truly durable and measurable definition of health is more than just a sound bite.

These new definitions lead to a corollary issue: "Where is health?" For me the answer is: "Health is an emergent state of the whole organism," which means that its description is to be found in the whole organism rather than just in its parts, something Aristotle intuited more than 2,000 years ago.

## Health's Intrinsic Value

As the definition of health varies, so too do the proclamations of its value. Herophilus asserted, "When health is absent, wisdom cannot reveal itself, art cannot become manifest, strength cannot fight, wealth becomes useless, and intelligence cannot be applied" (19). Hippocrates, not surprisingly, felt that "health is the most valuable possession" (20). Plato added, "Life without health is not worth living." (21) Huang-di, the emperor who laid the foundation for traditional Chinese medicine some 4,500 years ago, proclaimed that "protecting and developing health must rank even above that of restoring it when it is compromised" (22). Descartes claimed, "The preservation of health is without doubt the chief blessing of all the blessings in life" (23). Disraeli gave it a social context: "Health is the foundation on which rests the happiness of the people and the power of a country" (24). "The care of the public health is the first duty of a statesman." *Salvus populis supremus lex* (24A).

Yet despite this abundance of passionate testimonials to it, health, like Rodney Dangerfield, gets no respect. The word itself seems too bland. We are curious only about things that overtly affect our daily life. The transparency, the "given-ness" of health, limits commitment to our new mode of well-being, the new choice.

Beyond this, the word "health" itself has been misappropriated and has become a platitude. Health care, in the current nomenclature, is not really health care, but disease care. Health insurance is not health insurance, but disease insurance. Community health care centers are community disease care centers. The NHS and the NIH are effectively the NDS and NID. Yet collectively, we are more comfortable with the term "health," which encourages its misuse. We know vastly more about disease than we do about health, just as we tend to know more about why our car does not run than about why and how it does.

In his book *Unweaving the Rainbow,* Richard Dawkins describes John Keats's discomfort with Newton's scientific appraisal of a rainbow (25). In his poem "Lamia," Keats chided Newton for denigrating the ineffable beauty of a rainbow by reducing it to measurable units, the lengths of the various light waves. Dawkins and others since have risen to this challenge and responded that in fact, the rainbow achieves exalted beauty and splendor and importance by being knowable rather than by being merely sensed. I make this same claim for health.

With his new tools of mechanics, Newton worked hard to measure his domain (26). What are the angles? The forces? The spaces? The speed? Similarly, what are the measurements of the health domain? If we are to give health a new definition, it must be expressible in numbers; it must reveal its metrics. For the first time in history, we now have the necessary tools, data, and conceptual framework to put numbers on health's space, span, and pace.

## The Metrics of Life I: Health's Space

Health is fortunate to have much redundancy built into it. Most of nature's organs are paired, including the eyes, ears, lungs, kidneys, testicles, and ovaries. Any creature can perform its daily chores adequately with only one of these paired elements. This infers that given a birthright of 100% function, we can subtract 50% without risk to survival or severe impairment in overall function. Subtract another 10%, and we are down to 40% of starting allotment, and still no impairment appears. After another 10% loss, however, leaving only 30% of starting functional space, symptoms occur, such as blurring of vision, weakness, shortness of breath and the like. Another 10% loss, down to 20% of starting allotment, and profound functional impairment or death threatens.

This is easily grasped with regard to the paired organs, but it holds for a wide variety of actions. This general formulation is described in Figure 8.1. It is

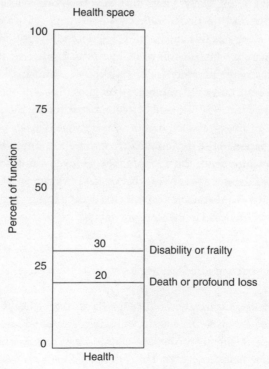

**Figure 8.1** Health space.

in the 20% to 30% of total health range that illness and its diagnosis, treatment, and costs all become apparent. The threshold value of 30% of total function applies to oxygen transport, myocardial oxygen consumption, arterial cross-sectional area, hemoglobin oxygen dissociation, maximum breathing capacity, forced expiratory volume, hematologic values, platelets, white blood cell count, prothrombin level, hepatic and renal function, blood sugar, sensory capacity (vision and hearing), cognitive skills, and brain dopamine content. Each exhibits approximately a 70% functional safety threshold. Other parameters such as red blood cell count and nerve conduction velocity show less redundancy. Muscle strength is another central function. In order to be able to walk, a person requires 1.2 watts per kilogram of energy quotient. The typical person possesses 5 watts per kilogram. Below 0.5 watts per kilogram, walking is impossible, which conforms to the above scale.

Such range has been recognized elsewhere. In a 1993 article, physiologist Pendergast and colleagues at the University of Buffalo consider 35% of composite function as being the lower boundary of adequate functionality (27). Gerontologist Verdery of the Aging Center, University of Arizona, calls the range between 20% and 40% "the survival range" (28). These estimates conform generally to the "safety factors" that Jared Diamond identified in a wide variety of structures and functions of different animal species, from squid to mammals (29). The teleology of this apparent "extra" function represents the organism's survival margin when environmental perturbations arise. It is interesting to note that this range of safety factors is also very similar to that specified by civil engineering codes for inanimate structures (30).

While the establishment of a core metric for the range of health is generally helpful, it must be noted that the upper range of health is not rigid. While the lower parameter of dysfunction (recognition of limitations or death) is set by stern requirements, the upper functional level, our potential, is highly dependent on adaptive capacity, or what we have previously referred to as phenotypic plasticity—the organism's capacity to adapt to reach maximum potential, which is always higher than the standard values.


## The Metrics of Life II: Lifespan

Having established the metrics for the space of health, we are prompted to examine its span. Once again, our exploration and knowledge of lifespan are still recent and surprisingly shallow. The Bible's Methuselah is certainly no reference help. And even Dr. Alexander Leaf's famous *National Geographic* article on the three supposedly super-geron populations of Hunza, in northeast

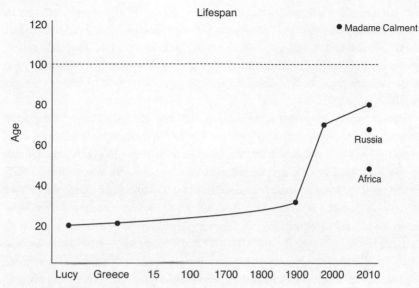

**Figure 8.2** Health span.

Pakistan, Georgia, and Vilcabamba, Ecuador, served only to delay our ability to gauge the human lifespan accurately (31).

The best evidence we have currently is the case of Madame Calment of Arles, France, who is documented to have lived 122 years (32). I have visited with her doctor, Dr. Jean-M. Robine, heard reports on her well-being at medical meetings until her death, and have a copy of her birth certificate in my desk drawer. She was frisky right up until she died. "I have only one wrinkle in my body, and I'm sitting on it," she is reported to have said. Dr. Robine has joined other sleuths in tracking the late-life courses of the "super-centenarians," individuals older than 110 years. As of February 2010, the Gerontology Research Group lists 75 such individuals worldwide, the oldest having been Gertrude Baines of Los Angeles, who was born April 6, 1894, and died on September 11, 2009. Undoubtedly there are many others who deserve to be on the list but so far have not "come out" (33).

We should note here that "lifespan" and "life expectancy" are not the same. The term "lifespan" is reserved for the species-specific, genetically ordained maximum life term of an organism, while life expectancy is always a fraction of that, as it represents the actual observed life duration, not the potential maximum. Whereas life expectancy generally trends upward, in some countries it has decreased. Lifespan, on the other hand, remains unchanged for many thousands of years: Lucy's lifespan and ours are likely the same.

The arena of interest that denotes the lifespan of a species continues to enlarge. A recent paper in *Physiological Reviews* identifies three major contributing elements to the lifespan of a species (34). First is that species' specific structure. Second is the effect of catabolic change, commonly attributed to the action of free radicals. And third is the possibility that these oxidative changes can be repaired.

The primary lifespan determinant is the rate-of-living theory, somewhat amended. This idea originated with the German physiologist Max Rubner in 1908 (35) and was elaborated by Raymond Pearl in 1928 (36). Stephen J. Gould, in *The Panda's Thumb,* stated that all animals live the same amount, but at different rates (37). All animals breathe about 200,000 times per lifetime and have 800,000 or so heartbeats. These are both derived from the common metabolic endowment of a fixed number of calories per kilogram per lifetime. Since all cells are made of the same stuff, CHNOPS, obey the same metabolic rules, and share the same temperature, which determines the rate of chemical reactions, we can expect that lifespan should be predictable. Even the way restricted feeding lengthens lifespan, first demonstrated by my father's associate Clive McCay at Cornell in the 1930s, seems to be easily reconciled with the rate-of-living theory (38).

But the theory requires substantial amendment to conform to the wide range of lifespans in the living world. The work of Dennis Harman is central to the free-radical theory of lifespan determination (39). Free radicals (discussed in more detail later) are the inevitable tax on life, the cost of living. Since metabolism generates trash, these free radicals, lifespan would seem to be intimately related to these metabolic terrorists. Birds, however, have high metabolic rates (or rates of energy transfer, also discussed later) and high levels of free radical production, but lifespans that seem uncommonly long. This is possibly due to their greater ability to sop up the free radicals through better repair. In another example, fruit flies that have high levels of free radical-neutralizing enzymes live longer (40,41).

The *Physiological Reviews* article encompasses wear-and-tear and repair, but also adds a third element of an organism's composition—unsaturated fatty acids—to the exponential equation used to derive lifespan (34). While the details of the weights of the different exponentials are being worked out, there is increasing agreement that human lifespan is potentially in the 120- to 130-year range. Ken Manton of Duke, our leading age demographer, asserts that an increasing number of people may live to 130 (42). Two prominent gerontologists, S. Jay Olshansky and Steve Austad, have a wager between them that even 130 is not the ultimate lifespan (43). Austad figures that further knowledge and technology will permit the imagination to range to even higher projections.

I am skeptical of this position because so far as I know there is no respite from the Second Law of Thermodynamics, which rules the human lifespan as it does all processes.

Meanwhile, life expectancy continues to increase unless, as Olshansky suggests, the current obesity and diabetes epidemics mean that a shortening of life expectancy may lie directly ahead (44). It is part of the mission of this book to see that this does not happen. For now, the operational term for the human health span is reasonably set at 120 years, or about 1 million hours. The middle of the relevant bell-shaped curve is 100 years. The challenge remains to live well long enough to reach this potential, which is precisely the goal of Next Medicine.

## The Metrics of Life III: Health's Pace

Next is health pace. How quickly do events occur? To set the proposition in terms for which data are available, it is important to select a starting date for health. The obvious alpha date point is conception, when sperm and egg come together, but we have only a dim glimpse of the details of early fetal health. Growing information indicates that the early intrauterine environment and its interaction with the fetus probably have lifelong effects (45). Studies of the life histories of babies born to women who were pregnant in periods of severe caloric shortage reveal critical changes that can be ascribed to suboptimal early nutrition (46).

After birth, the anabolic processes of development and growth are mixed with the catabolic reactions of life, so that it is hard to differentiate between the two. After growth is completed, however, let us say around 20 years of age, clear functional parameters, such as maximum pulse rate, emerge and can be accurately measured. We know that there is a set number of times the heart can beat per minute, depending upon a subject's age. The common formula for maximum heart rate is 220 minus your age. Similarly, structural elements of the body, such as bone and muscle strength and skin elasticity, show age-related loss.

In trying to determine the basic rate of change in humans, my physician son Walter and I surveyed the performances of competitive rowers, swimmers, and runners. When we plotted their results against age, we found a similar rate of decline of 0.5% per year for all events, as seen in Figure 8.3 (47). It is our contention that this figure presents the actual rate of age-related change, as these results represent the participation of every part of the body, from head to toe. Invoking the principle of symmorphosis, we contend that if any single part of the body were to deteriorate at a rate faster than 0.5% per year, that altered

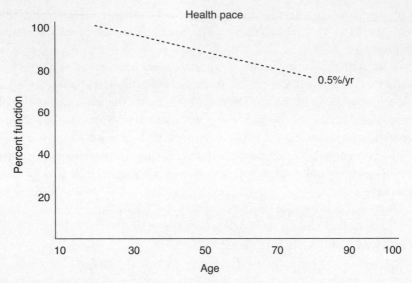

**Figure 8.3** Health pace.

parameter would become rate limiting. In other words, the body lasts only as long as its most precarious part. We published these results in our 1996 article in the *Journal of Gerontology,* "How Fast Do We Age?" and assert that 0.5% per year is the true base rate of life and health pace. F. E. Yates and Mary Sehl of the UCLA School of Medicine expanded on our original paper, looking at 445 separate studies and 13 different organ functions, and confirmed the rate of 0.5% per year (48). This rate is graceful, and not especially observable over a short period of time. We assert that any decrease in health pace that exceeds 0.5% per year is not due to aging; another cause should be sought. If, however, we plot this decay in rate against the above health pace, we see that the level at which we become aware of diminished health pace—30%—is not encountered until 150 years of age.

To explain this inconsistency, we project that the rate of 0.5% per year holds only for that period for which there are adequate data—that is, until approximately 70 years of age (49). It seems to us that until this age all body systems participate in parallel at the 0.5% rate. When one component deteriorates faster than 0.5% per year, it becomes deterministic and a cascade of other failures, replacing the 0.5% rate with a crescendo, leads to failure before the age of 150. In an as-yet-unpublished article, Gene Yates and Steve Pincus have proposed the above cascade to reconcile this hypothesis with observed longevity records (49).

## The Determinants of Health

Until recent history, human health was ruled largely by fate, but we now have the knowledge to replace fate with choice. The immediate questions that arise are: To what extent can we choose to be healthy? What determines health?

There has been very little systematic and comprehensive inquiry into this critical issue of health determinants. As a medical student, I was instructed (as thousands, maybe millions, before and since) that health is a byproduct of three interacting elements: host, agent, and environment. This disease-centric triad, largely an extrapolation from the millions of illnesses caused by infection, continues to be a core precept of the public health system. Thoughtful people, however, have recognized the severe limitations of this definition of health determinants. Most have concluded that health has a much broader cultural context than biology alone, and that non-biological factors such as education and economics have a significant effect on individual and public health. Millions of words have been uttered and written on non-biological health determinants. For example, most of the March 2002 issue of *Health Affairs*, the leading health policy journal, was devoted to this subject (50). Almost all the articles in the issue dealt with the many social and economic factors that affect health. The important document *Healthy People 2010* presents a summary scheme, shown in Figure 8.4. The figure shows that biology, behavior, physical environment, and social environment have roughly equal impacts on health.

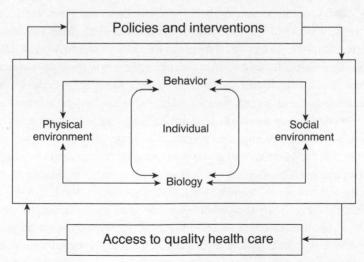

**Figure 8.4** Determinants of health. From "Healthy People 2010: Understanding and Improving Health," US Department of Health and Human Services, Washington, DC, 2000.

I am as aware of the importance of these forces to health as anyone, but I believe that the more immediate determinants are found in the biological aspects of health. Poor education and living conditions, poor atmosphere, and so on have strong correlations with health markers, but the direct biological events that occur to the human body ultimately determine health (51). Further, my medical school-era rubric of host, agent, and environment fails to include the roles played by genes and aging in the phenotypic health profile; these simply were not on the radar screen then.

To rectify the omission of the alpha and omega life features in the earlier formulation, I have proposed a new schematic with four discrete agencies. The metaphor of car health helps here. The life of a car depends on four elements: design, accidents, maintenance, and aging. If the car is a lemon, is involved in a major accident, or is poorly maintained, it will not have the chance to grow old. The same four categories apply to the human organism, but are more appropriately designated genes, external agency, internal agency, and aging. I propose that these four factors, occurring in innumerable combinations and chronologies, account for the totality of the human health experience, both individual and collective. Hypothetically, if the first three of these four factors could be eliminated through a perfect design or gene set, no accidents or external disruptions, and ideal maintenance or balanced internal dynamics, then the car—or we—would have the opportunity to die of natural causes, of aging.

Before I get into each of the four agents that determine health, let's make the connection between the key science topics of the previous chapter, some of the metrics above, and these determinants of health. Every cell at rest carries on its basal activity while idling. But this baseline functioning does not represent even a bare survival enterprise, as nature is constantly scrutinizing (in Darwin's phrase) all energetic challenges. All of the cell's hundreds to thousands of receptor sites are continually scanning the environment for energy cues—chemical, thermal, mechanical, electrical, and magnetic—that initiate a repertoire of cellular reactions, functional and structural. The genes listen in to this cueing, and turn on or off according to their script. Too many or too few signals do not serve the cell, but just the right amount of energetic stimulation maintains the cell's competence. The Golden Mean prevails. Figure 8.5 represents this "not too little, not too much" agenda of all cells. This figure, first drawn by Gene Yates on a paper napkin at breakfast one day, specifies the anabolic/catabolic (the two sides of metabolism—one building molecules and one breaking them down) effect of an energy flow on our tissues (52). An energetic stimulus will get a structural response if each link in the chain is working. Multiple gene complexes serving a variety of uses are at their functional optimum at a certain

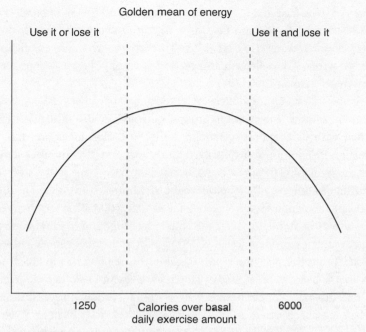

**Figure 8.5**  Golden mean of energy.

energetic range. This maximum potential, when achieved, is good health, good performance, and occasionally gold medals.

This level is plastic. It has distinct parameters that can be quantified. The gene cartels, through homeodynamic processes, obey deterministic energetic principles. The whole organism performs best when the metabolism and the genes are integrated and harmonious. This is health, the emergent state of the entire organism, when all the sub- compartments are optimally tuned to the specifications contained within the guidelines of the human potential. Now, on to the individual determinants of health.

## Genes

The history, structure, and function of the gene are by now well researched and archived. What largely remains is understanding precisely how important genes are to our health. The public acclaim accompanying the Human Genome Project, "genomania," led enthusiasts to proclaim that genes, when fully under-stood, would lead to complete computation of the organism. This assumption has proved to be false and misleading, much to the detriment of public aware-ness of gene science. Richard Lewontin, in *Not in Our Genes*, asserts the bad biology of such claims (53). M. J. West-Eberhard, who studies phenotypic plasticity, wrote, "The sole gene in isolation is among the most impotent and useless material imaginable" (54).

We now know a critical dimension of the gene story: that genes are far from aloof in their tasks. They work in groups, networks, which in turn are closely matched with biochemical metabolic complexes. Hormones are important modulators. Genes are functionally de-localized and structurally entangled. Genes are plastic and dynamic. Dawkins used the term "gene cartel" to describe their group significance (55), and Barbara McClintock's investigations discov-ered the phenomenon of gene flux, or gene mobility (56). They are often redun-dant, so that the notion of one gene equals one function is simply not valid, though it remains a widely accepted connection in the public imagination.

Some projections cite thousands of genes that are involved in the structure of an eye, a heart, a brain, and so forth. A reductionistic depiction of one gene/one disease has now been largely eclipsed. Although several thousand single-gene–caused diseases have now been identified, Richard Strohman, University of California Berkeley emeritus professor of biology, has estimated that less than 2% of all human illness is due to a faulty single-gene locus (57). Far more commonly, complexity reigns. It is said that even an identified genetic disease such as cystic fibrosis has 350 different gene profiles in its description. Think of the gene not as an independent agent, but as one that plays a partici-pating role in homeodynamic processes, which mediates the transformation of energy into structure. The gene is constantly cued. It is variably expressed, and it is in these myriad complex expression patterns that the operational features reside. Genes act less as on/off switches than as rheostats with variable respon-sivity. Epigenetics, the study of the gene and its environment, is the new "hot field," the new "epicenter" for medicine, in Johns Hopkins physician Andrew Feinberg's term (58).

Undoubtedly a large part of the stridency and overreaching of the gene dogma was driven by commercial aspiration. In 2005, there were over 5,000 gene patents in effect, each representing fortune if not fame to the patent holder. Attempts to finger a particular gene for social problems (compulsive shopping, for instance) have further diminished the prestige and value of the single-gene emphasis. Genes have been sharply circumscribed in their importance as single health determinants.

An approach widely used to quantify genetic contributions is to investigate the health history of identical twins. If genes were ultimately determinative, and the other three agencies were only negligible factors in assuring health, then identical twins would die simultaneously of the same disease. This is far from the actual case (45). Common neurological diseases of older people (Parkinson's and Alzheimer's) have been shown to have low or no concordance among twins (59). Further studies of mono- and dizygotic twins indicate that heredity accounts for 15% to 20% of the differences in human longevity. Malcolm Zaretsky, who reviewed the case histories retained in the Institute of Medicine of World War II male twin survivors, casts some doubt even on this similarity (60). Zaretsky showed a similar degree of correlation with longevity, but when he looked more closely he found that much of the seeming coincidence was not due to genetics as much as it was to social bonding mechanisms. In summary, the twin data led to the simple homily, "It's not the cards you're dealt so much as how you play your hand."

## Accidents: External Agency

I define *accidents* as those situations in which the car or we are blithely going about our business when an unexpected and unavoidable event occurs; another car runs a stop sign, or a malevolent virus invades our body. The car, or person, was previously intact, but that state is disrupted by the assault of an external force.

Throughout history, the major threat to human health has arisen from an adverse encounter with a hostile force. Pasteur demonstrated that equating sickness with some sort of metaphysical punishment was wrong (61); the real devil was the microbe. The appropriate response to this new reality was to construct a therapeutic armor to shield the unsuspecting host from his or her dangerous environment.

The variety of health threats that the external world presents is immense. Injury, infection, toxins, and malignancy each blindside the human population every day. These threats may diminish the health reserve catastrophically, or they may conspire to build up trivial or sequential insults. For the most part they are acute in presentation and are usually confined to a defect in one body part.

In my opinion, the conditions involved in the external agency category are responsible for the development of most of the current medical enterprise of hospitals, surgery, technology, and pharmacy. Medical science has gained gaudy credentials by confronting the conditions secondary to faulty external agency. Technical advances have allowed us to address and redress countless illness states that were unapproachable just a few decades ago.

In addition, the issue of prevention arises when we consider defining external agency as a health determinant. Most infections, injuries, and malignancies are

preventable, and preventing them is a strategy far preferable to curing them—
and cheaper. To paraphrase Oliver Wendell Holmes, "The shield is nobler than
the spear" (62).

## Maintenance: Internal Agency

Disordered internal functioning has replaced external agents as the principal
cause of the chronic illness patterns we see today. These internal conditions
tend to involve the entire system rather than merely certain components, as
in external agency problems. Instead of the environment being a threat to
well-being, internal agency connotes an appropriate and constant interplay
between host and environment. The environment becomes a source of organic
order and stability and therefore of health maintenance, a central point in Ilya
Prigogine's *Order Out of Chaos* (63). The car, for instance, has two principal
maintenance elements: fuel and engine speed. Too little or too much fuel, or
bad fuel, can compromise your car's functioning. So, too, if you run the car too
hard or not hard enough, it will end up in the repair shop.

I have previously described the very severe threat that we now encounter,
the result not of genes or external agency or aging, but of the faulty mechanisms
of internal agency. Key to internal agency is our concept of the body's total
energy balance and flow. The effects of taking in more energy than we use are
profound—homeodynamics, plasticity, and symmorphosis see to it. But first,
let us start with one of our intakes—oxygen.

The importance of oxygen to health has been known since ancient times.
The ancients spoke of "the breath of life." Oxygen drives life, which is health.
Science is capable of measuring the organism's capacity to use oxygen. This
measurement is usually done in exercise physiology labs, and its specific term
is $Vo_2$ max. It is generally considered the best indicator of cardiorespiratory fitness and aerobic fitness. $Vo_2$ max simply represents the measured ability of the
organism to transport oxygen through all its respiratory conduits, eventually to
the mitochondria, where energy is generated.

$Vo_2$ max can be measured in the clinic by putting the subject on a treadmill
or a bike and providing him or her with a specific amount of oxygen, then
monitoring to determine the maximum intake. In this sense, it is a measure of
a body's capacity to use oxygen as fuel. The response to the amount of physical
exercise is corollary. Exercise is often expressed as the amount of oxygen consumed per minute per kilogram. For humans, resting values are approximately
3.5 mL per kilogram per minute. The highest exercise value recorded was that
of a cross-country skier: 94 mL per kilogram per minute, a 27-fold increase

above baseline. Racehorses increase their metabolic rate 45-fold over baseline, but like the skier, such usage can be sustained only for short periods, as in sprinting. The highest sustained oxygen consumption was measured in four cyclists in the 1984 Tour de France. For the 2 weeks and 3,826 km of extreme exertion, the riders averaged 5,900 cal per day, which is 4.3 times higher than the resting rate, with no change in body mass (64). An average sedentary person expends 1.7 times basal usage in ordinary activities; a coal miner expends 2.5 times basal. Therefore, oxygen/calorie consumption is highly dependent on the environmental energy challenge.

Such oxygen-using capacity reflects the environmental imprinting on function-phenotypic plasticity at work. As we plot $Vo_2$ max in fit persons, we observe the 0.5% decline as expected. But Drs. F. Kasch and J. L. Boyer of San Diego showed that unfit people's $Vo_2$ max declines at 2% per year (65) (Fig. 8.6). The takeaway message of these critical data is that a fit person of 70 has the oxygen delivery capacity of an unfit 40-year-old. Fitness, therefore, is a 30-year age offset. The implication is profound: you can't do anything about the 0.5% slope, but you can tackle the 2% slope, just not with anything found in a drugstore.

Our second major intake is, of course, food. Our entire evolutionary history was shaped by ensuring caloric sufficiency. Most early people, like most animals, starved to death. In the blink of an eye, this reality has been overcompensated by caloric surfeit. For the first time in the history of the human species, we

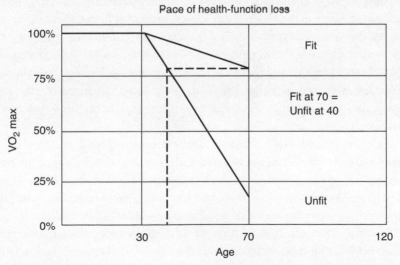

**Figure 8.6** $Vo_2$ max/fitness. From "Physical Fitness and All-Cause Mortality," *Journal of the American Medical Association,* November 3, 1989, Volume 262, page 2396. Copyright © 1989, American Medical Association. All rights reserved.

have more overweight than underweight people on the globe, according to a recent WHO study (66). In 2004, *National Geographic* headlined obesity as an international threat, coining the term *globesity* (67). I spent the early part of my investigative career fixating on problems of fat metabolism and received a large multiyear NIH grant for a study titled "The Effect of Diet on the Metabolism of Fat in Man," from which dozens of papers and several textbook chapters on obesity resulted (68).

The surge in contemporary obesity rates looks like a contagion. A generation ago, fat children were relatively rare; now they are common and even, in many places, the norm. Largely because of this surge, the Centers for Disease Control and Prevention (CDC) has acknowledged that we may be seeing the first generation of Americans since the nation's founding who could have a shorter life expectancy than their parents.

An insistent aspect of the nutritional component of our maintenance is inappropriate energetic stimulation. This maladaptation becomes increasingly important as we age. Misapplied energy comes in two forms: too much and too little. Too much energetic interfacing is known by the term "stress" and too little is known as "disuse." Both have vast negative consequences on the affected organism, and both are inadequately recognized as basic health threats. Part of the reason for this is the long timeline from cause to effect.

Eminent McGill University endocrinologist Hans Selye was the first to describe the spectrum of stressors that assault organisms. He labeled the host response to these challenges the "general adaptation syndrome" (69). Bruce McEwen, director of the Neuroendocrine Laboratory at Rockefeller University, coined the term *allostatic load* to quantify the cumulative physiological toll exerted on the body over time by efforts to adapt to life experience (70). A 1997 report in the *Archives of Internal Medicine* by Theresa Seeman and colleagues indicated that allostatic load was a better predictor of cognitive decline and cardiovascular performance in older people than more standard parameters (71).

The converse of stress is disuse. Disuse means too little energetic interchange, usually manifested in a sedentary lifestyle. Figure 8.5 showed the relationship between healthy fitness levels and energy throughput (energy used). Clearly, total energy increases as activity levels increase. The figure shows that there is a requisite minimum range of activity—about 2,500 kilocalories per week above a bed rest, "idling," amount. Too little activity and anabolic yield (the processes that build molecules, cells, and tissues) is low; too much activity and anabolic yield is also lowered (cells and tissues need repair from overuse). So, at one end of the activity scale, "use it *or* lose it" applies, and at the other end "use it *and* lose it" applies. The Golden Mean is the Golden Range.

I codified the common clinical parameters within the rubric of "the disuse syndrome": cardiovascular vulnerability, musculoskeletal fragility, immunological susceptibility, metabolic instability, central nervous system risk, frailty, and precocious aging (72). Each of these components has distinct deterministic mechanisms that relate insufficient energetic throughput to the frequently observed disease byproducts. These are not genetic or externally produced, nor are they secondary to aging *per se*. Instead, they are the explicit byproducts of protracted disuse. My rubric of the disuse syndrome was anticipated by Hans Krause and Wilhelm Raab in 1961 as "hypokinetic disease" (73). The "sedentary death syndrome" similarly codified by Frank Booth also connects our collective descent into sedentary lifestyles to the pathologies of our time (74). Data from the Bureau of Economic Research indicate that workers who spend their careers in a sedentary job have a BMI (body mass index) 3.3 units higher than those in active jobs (75). This difference is equivalent to the weight that has been gained across the population during the last 100 years. Stanford's noted childhood obesity expert Tom Robinson estimates that 25% of Americans' waking hours are spent watching TV, which is bad enough, but 20% of the daily calories are consumed while sitting in front of the TV screen (76). Numerous studies indicate a 20% to 30% daily deficit of physical activity. Only 28% of the students of Santa Clara, California, passed a simple fitness evaluation (77).

James Levine at the Mayo Clinic has hypothesized that non-exercise activity thermogenesis (NEAT) is a major contributor to our total caloric expenditure, though it is generally overlooked or unspecified (78)—in other words, our caloric expenditure when we are not engaged in exercise. Fidgeting is one example of this. Quantitative estimates record that this workaday component of caloric usage is even higher than the identified exercise expenditure. It ranges from 15% of total energy expenditure to over 50%, depending on the particular activity. Levine feels that our societal slothfulness is mostly attributable to non-occupational lifestyle features such as the car, TV, video games, elevators and escalators, remote control devices, vicarious exercise, and dishwashers, to name a few. My particular villain is the golf cart, as I am an ardent golfer given the opportunity. Golf to me is a wonderful walk in a beautiful setting interrupted by periodic missed shots. But now golf is a ride and barely qualifies as exercise.

The central role that physical inactivity plays in regulating total body energy balance and therefore the odds of getting or not getting obese or diabetic cannot be overemphasized. Every study indicates that we are moving less and less: fewer than 40% of Americans are even minimally physically active (79). This inactivity plays no age favorites: both kids and oldsters sit too much. I spent much of my professional career asserting that many of the changes, including the upward trend in diabetes incidence, that are commonly attributed to aging *per se* are in reality due to the increased sitting time that older people defer to. Inactivity can be deadly.

Multiplying all these opportunities for "least effort" more than qualifies as the major contributor to our obesity epidemic. A *British Medical Journal* editorial in 1995 asked "Obesity: gluttony or sloth?" and concluded that sloth was the larger perpetrator (80). A National Bureau of Economic Research report reached a similar conclusion (75).

Symmorphosis is the central concept in understanding this phenomenon. This newly established unifying feature of physiology explains why all parts of a functional network operate in parallel. Symmorphosis explains why the lack of physical exertion underlies fully 50% of our clinical profiles, as our genes are miscued by our habit of disuse. Through symmorphosis, the linked systemic effects of decreased energy flow are inscribed onto the human health agenda. What remains to be discussed is how much and to what extent.

The internal agency factor of physical fitness looms large when we consider the spectrum of clinical conditions ascribable to the disuse syndrome. Steven Blair, former director of research at Cooper Clinic in Dallas, was the principal author of the Surgeon General's report on physical exercise in 1996 (81). While at Cooper, Dr. Blair wrote what I consider to be the second most important paper in the past 50 years of medical science, "Physical Fitness and All-cause Mortality: A prospective Study of Healthy Men and Women," published in *JAMA* in 1989 (82). Blair reviewed 13,344 participants, people who had undergone a preventive medical screening examination at the Cooper Clinic. As part of the exam, they underwent an exercise electrocardiogram and other lab tests. The treadmill tests provided an objective measure of cardiorespiratory fitness. Over the 8 years of observation, there were 283 deaths. There was a three- to four-fold difference in mortality rates between the least and most fit groups, and this difference increased markedly with age.

Blair's group recently updated its earlier report (83). In this study they looked at 2,603 individuals over age 60 for a period of 12 years. There were 450 deaths, and the protective benefits of fitness described in the initial study were affirmed. It is incontestable that the older we grow, the more important fitness becomes (Fig. 8.7). For men over 60, the higher the fitness category, the lower the mortality rate. The saying should not be, "you are too old to exercise." Instead, it should be, "you are too old *not* to exercise." Maria Fiatarone's classic paper in *JAMA* a few years back wonderfully showed that feeble, "noodle-legged" 90-year-old nursing home residents reacted briskly to an exercise protocol (84). It is not necessarily exercise as commonly conceived in the context of a gym or competitive sport activity, but rather the energetics supplied by a

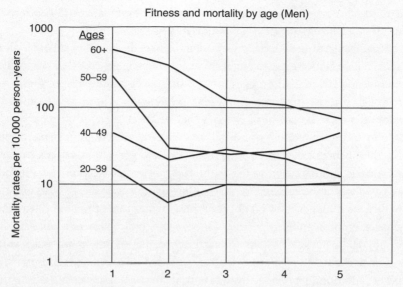

**Figure 8.7** Vo$_2$ max/age. From "Physical Fitness and All Causes of Mortality," *Journal of the American Medical Association,* November 3, 1989, Volume 262, page 2396. Copyright © 1989, American Medical Association. All rights reserved.

physically active lifestyle that exert strong homeodynamic, symmorphotic effects on all the body organs and functions that sustain life.

Numerous large observational studies address the inactivity/obesity/diabetes/ mortality axes. The recent statistics on children are even more startling than the ones on adults. There has been a shocking 10-fold increase in type II diabetes in children in the 12-year period between 1982 and 1994 (85). The inactivity/ obesity/diabetes connection is crucial. An 8-year review of 70,000 nurses revealed 1,419 new cases of diabetes, and the more fit nurses had half the incidence of diabetes of the less fit ones (86). The ongoing Physicians' Health Study of 21,271 doctors, begun in 1982, revealed a 5-year incidence of new diabetes of 285, with fitness once again providing a 50% protection factor (87). In a Cooper Aerobic Center review of 2,196 diabetics, 275 died during a 15-year observation period; the difference in death rate between the most and least fit was 1:4.5 (88). Another Cooper study showed that unfit men were four times as likely to become diabetic as fit men. A large survey of 34,257 women in Minnesota revealed that *any* amount of physical activity lowered the incidence of new diabetes by 30%. A study in Malmo, Sweden, reviewed the life histories of a group of people with prediabetes and found that an exercise intervention lowered their mortality rate to that of persons who were not prediabetic (89). Exercise "cured" prediabetes, at least as far as mortality was concerned.

These results directly and indirectly demonstrate the great benefit of physical activity. These facts are key to establishing a strong science-based public-policy recommendation that encourages those with budget-making responsibility to put a high priority on encouraging physical activity. When we dig down to explore the basic biochemical changes that occur as a result of exercise, we come to an understanding of how all the wide-ranging body benefits occur, since the biochemical changes triggered by exercise pervade all tissues, organs, and systems. Fundamental to this is the fact that exercise represents a higher rate of energy transfer. Exercise makes the engine run faster. You might ask whether these higher rates do not result in a higher rate of wear and tear and the generation of more trash, such as those free radicals. Aren't you actually consuming the number of lifetime heartbeats while running uphill, when your pulse may reach 140 or higher? True enough, but as a result of the improved level of conditioning provided by hill running, the resting pulse rate falls to the 40s, in contrast to the "norm" of 72 in unconditioned persons. Thus the net number of heartbeats in conditioned hill runners is less than the number of beats in the sedentary individual.

Similarly, the amount of free radicals generated during exercise is elevated, but the increase is more than compensated for by the higher levels of the scavenging enzymes that consume the radicals as they form (90). The net effect of a conditioning program is to lessen the mischief that these "molecular terrorists" do.


## Aging

We now come to our fourth and final determinant of health: aging. Largely unrecognized in the rush of high-profile science breakthroughs is the fact that we now have enough data about the basic biological reality of aging to create a useful conceptual framework of that process. Too often in the past, the aged have been presented as caricatures. King Lear, "that ruined piece of nature," and Ponce de Leon represent sad remnants of life. Of course, part of the reason for the shortage of positive views of aging is the fact that aging has been a rarity, both in animals and in early humans. There were occasional old individuals, but they were exceptional and usually considered outliers. But the globe now fully recognizes the Methuselah phenomenon, which is affecting the whole world, challenging and upsetting old norms and values and economies.

We need an exploration of the biology of growing old. Invoking the principle of emergence, is it appropriate to ask: At which organizational level of the organism does aging occur? Aging, like life, is more than atoms and molecules. It is more than physics and chemistry, and we can apply the principle of emergence to aging, as we do to the function of life.

Ninety-seven years ago, the French biologist Alexis Carrel won a Nobel Prize for demonstrating that cells grown in isolation are immortal (91). This would presume that aging does not apply at the cellular level. Unfortunately, Carrell was wrong. In 1962, Leonard Hayflick showed conclusively that cells carefully nurtured in cell culture plates have a finite lifespan (92). They have only so many reproductive doublings available to them before they die; this finding is now known as the Hayflick limit. The intracellular details of this programmed aging are still under review as of this writing, but we can assume that aging is inevitable and natural.

In the attempt to understand aging, it is essential that we broaden the inquiry beyond the living world, because everything in the universe ages, including stars, canyons, Chevrolets, and tennis shoes. Further, aging has a unidirectional time factor inherent in it, the "arrow of time." Aging, like time, is irreversible. Where do we go to find the universal law that embraces energy, matter, and time? Once again, it is the potent Second Law of Thermodynamics. My definition of aging, therefore, is the effect of an energy flow on matter over time. We must recall that this energy flow is ordering as well as disordering, so that the net effect, ordering minus disordering, equals aging.

The study of aging has been confused by the fact that the effects of other processes, such as deterioration due to external or internal agencies, have been included within its parameters. The frequently cited figure tracing the progressive, supposedly age-related declines in many body systems prepared by Nathan Shock in 1960 from the participants in the Baltimore Longitudinal Study has been shown to be fundamentally flawed, because inadvertently included in the study were diseased individuals, whose deficits were therefore wrongly attributed to age (93). The referenced figures of Sehl, Yates (48), and myself (47), which reflect the inclusive figure of a 0.5% decline per year, are held to be more representative of real age change. But there still has been no recorded instance of reversal of real age changes. This is not to say, however, that older individuals' functions inevitably get progressively worse. However, any seeming improvements are secondary to the capture of previously unrealized phenotypic potential. Importantly, age does not even serve as a disqualification of phenotypic improvement, leading to one of my favorite maxims, "It's never too late to start, but it's always too soon to stop."

Instead of being an inscrutable example of nature's fatigue, aging now stands revealed with rigorous defining parameters. "Aging is no longer an unknown," Hayflick wrote in the scientific journal PLoS in 2009 (94). Aging is a part of life.

I treasure my father's response to the challenge: "Dr. Bortz, how do you stop aging?" His answer, "I'm not interested in arrested development." If you are lucky or smart, then you will get to be old someday, which, as has been frequently observed, surely beats the alternative.

If there are going to be 1 billion people in the world over the age of 65 in 2060, some 330 million in China alone, we had better get with the program. Animals seldom have the chance to grow old in the wild, so we humans are the study organism. One of the central tasks in shifting medicine from a disease mode to a health mode is reformulating the process of aging. Having established the credentials of thermodynamics in providing a conceptual framework for life and health, we now invoke it in a rigorous approach to aging. Aging, like life, involves the three parameters of matter, energy, and time. Aging is tightly bound to metabolic processes, and as such it demonstrates the important quality of plasticity.

Using $Vo_2$ max as an important and instructive example, true age change predicts that the average person will experience a 0.5%-per-year decline. However, if insufficient energy is supplied, this rate can be 2% or more per year. More important, $Vo_2$ values of older, unfit individuals can be improved with an exercise protocol. Herbert DeVries's work at the University of Southern California indicates a potential recapture of 30 years' worth of apparent age change by a conditioning program provided to 70-year-olds: their $Vo_2$ improved to the levels of inactive 30-year-olds (95).

I have often used the following analogy: "Your grandfather clock stops running. The various diagnoses are: one, it is broken; two, it is worn out, or three, it needs to be wound up again" (96). Being broken fits the standard disease model of medicine, in which recourse to the repair shop is the appropriate next step. Being worn out is a reflection of true chronological decay. This is not susceptible to repair; the junkyard's the best option. But the third possibility, needing to be wound up, is an underrecognized alternative explanation. This is particularly important because winding up is cheap and doable and has no side effects. Too often, when confronted with a clock or a body that does not work as it should, we lapse into a disease inference—fix it, or cut it out, solder it, or replace it—rather than the appropriate approach, which is to let energy restore matter to its entitled state. Importantly, you cannot substitute surgery or pharmaceuticals or technical approaches for winding up. There simply is no proxy for energy. "Medicated survival," is how René Dubos termed our tendency to seek medical help when we cannot wind a wound-down organism. It is, after all, not how old you are that matters, but how you are old.

I was distressed by the approach advocated in influential circles and represented by the popular 2004 book *Coping with Methuselah* (97). This multi-authored volume provides a provocative look into a near future in which lifespans are extended considerably, but largely through a hypothetical fix of high technology, gene science, cloning, stem cells, and further developments in molecular biology. My perspective is that New Age wizardry will have little impact on aging, which is a stern expression of the Second Law of Thermodynamics from which there is no respite.

Age has been held to be the cause of too much late-life difficulty. My message is that this can be reversed through phenotypic plasticity if older people resume fitness regimens. The facile division of older people into usual and successful, Jack Rowe's and Bob Kahn's effort to identify "superior" older people in an influential 1987 article in *Science* (98), conceals the fact that usual can become successful by simple, safe, and cheap effort. What drug can make that assertion?

## Putting It All Together: The Health Equation

I have now identified and quantified each of the four biological determinants of health. Now it is time to combine them into a unified statement, a health equation:

$$\text{Genes (A) + Extrinsic Agency (B) + Intrinsic Agency (C) +}$$
$$\text{Aging (D) = Health}$$

Of course, plugging in the values of A, B, C, and D is the challenge. Let's make some assumptions and take that challenge:

A. Presuming lifespan to represent health, we obtain a 15% contribution of genes to longevity, and enter 0.15 as the coefficient for genes.
B. The extrinsic determinant can be anything, depending on the spin of the wheel; it can be catastrophic or zero. Presuming that life has not burdened us with catastrophes, B will be zero.
D. Aging 0.5% per year for an 80-year-old person might yield a 30% factor. Therefore, D equals 0.3.

Thus, we have 0.15 + 0 + intrinsic agency + 0.3 = Health

Or, combining factors, Health = 0.45 + intrinsic agency.

Intrinsic Agency = Health – 0.45

In other words, such reckoning, though admittedly coarse, means that internal agency accounts for around 55% of the values we need for health, which is similar to the figure obtained by Mike McGinnis of the Institute of

Medicine and Bill Foege of the Gates Foundation (99). More than half of all health issues are attributable to lifestyle and specific behaviors.

One of my prime reasons for proposing my scheme for the biological determinants of health was to encourage an objective categorization scheme for which a rational approach is possible. I am a fierce devotee of what is commonly called the Serenity Prayer, which I paraphrase as, "Change what you can, accept what you must, but know the difference" (100). My scheme specifically targets the difference. Factors A and D, the bookends to life, are rigidly coded in cosmic law and thus exempted from meaningful change. This leaves B and C, external and internal agency, as practical, "change what you can" goals for prevention and treatment. Injuries, infections, and even many cancers are probably preventable, so this strategy looms large.

When we solve the equation, internal agency (largely nutrition and physical fitness) emerges as the prime focus. Behavior can be changed. Natural law may deny our intervention, but nurture is amenable to amendment.

Having developed a new insight into what determines health, and recognizing the deficiencies inherent in the traditional causes of illness and death, mandates a fresh look at how we categorize. McGinnis and Foege's critical 1993 *JAMA* article, "Actual Causes of Death in the United States" (99), outlines the challenge inherent in this new recognition. Most death certificate entries are wrong; I know, because I have contributed a disproportionate number of them. We need a new taxonomy that encompasses time and system in its scope. If the actual cause of illness and death is a reflection of an inappropriate relationship between the organism and its environment, we need a way of capturing this in our labels. For better or for worse, the shorthand allocation of resources follows simple labels. But what if lung cancer, diabetes, heart disease, stroke, and the other common afflictions are not so simple, and so localized in their identity? What if these pathologies are really the end products of inappropriate symmorphotic and homeodynamic energetic interplay between the organism and its environment? What shall I put down on my required diagnostic forms? It generates a smile when I consider the reaction of the clerk who receives such a polysyllabic new taxonomy.

So as we transition from Disease Medicine to Health Medicine and from Current Medicine to Next Medicine, we have new definitions, new metrics, new determinants, and a new taxonomy to incorporate. Accomplishing this will be a challenge, but its implementation will evolve in pace with the new operational schemes that Next Medicine will generate.

Health is unwoven. We newly know ourselves. We can assert our potential. Our nature is revealed. Now then, how best to nurture it?

# Tons to Ounces—Repair to | 9
# Prevention

Prevention has been severely devalued as a main pillar of our effort to assure the human potential, but Next Medicine puts it front and center in our daily lives. Prevention can no longer be a bland platitude, but must become the centerpiece of our conception of health.

Although we have all heard that an ounce of prevention is worth a pound of cure millions of times, this has not really been our practice. Twenty-five years ago, Anne Somers, former professor of public health at Rutgers University, wrote a terse article in the *New England Journal of Medicine* entitled "Why Not Try Preventing Illness as a Way of Controlling Medicare Costs?" (1). Lamenting the "blind spot in U.S. health policy," she quoted the president of the Association of Life Insurance Medical Directors of America: "We all know there is no single answer, nor a quick fix, and the more we tamper with some aspects of the problem the more we aggravate others. The only logical way to go is prevention." In a 2006 perspective in *Health Affairs*, "The Prevention Challenge and Opportunity," David Satcher advocated strongly for a prevention strategy, and observed that less than 2% of our health budget is allocated to it (2).

At a regional meeting of the Institute of Medicine of the National Academy of Sciences in San Francisco on November 17, 2009, Harvey Feinberg reported in his president's address that "the current debate on the future of health care in our country, rather than representing a single culminating act, is a progressive

139

sequential transformation that will play out over a period of years and be expressed in legislation, regulatory, scientific, technological, cultural, institutional, professional, educational, and ultimately social change." From this shopping list, he continues, "I begin with prevention, since it is so fundamental, and yet it is typically treated as an afterthought in health reform debate" (3).

Feinberg cited the fact that 300,000 fewer smokers light up in New York City than 7 years previously as the result of a broad-based strategy involving many components of the Big Apple. Overseeing this conversion to a systems approach was Tom Friedan, then New York City Commissioner of Health and now director of the CDC.

Supportive of this commitment to return to a preventive philosophy is $1.1 billion in funding from the economic stimulus package devoted to finding out which of the hosts of traditional medical repair strategies work and which do not. Such effort goes under the term of *comparative effectiveness research*. Feinberg finds much promise in this research.

The test case for this effort is prostate cancer. There are 200,000 new cases per year. The researchers reviewed 700 studies in which one of four treatment options was used: surgery, radiation, hormone chemotherapy, and watchful waiting. It was reported in the November 27, 2009, issue of *Science* that surgeons advised surgery, radiologists advised radiation, and oncologists advised chemotherapy (4). Very few advised watchful waiting. After a number of years, the results revealed that there was no difference in clinical outcome between the aggressive and conservative approach to treatment, despite huge differences in cost, time, and effort. The implications of this revelation shake the medical foundations to their base. How to know what to do? Repair where powerful advocates argue, or prevention whose proponents are muted?

Even in the most obvious conditions, such as AIDS, the fulcrum is sternly tilted toward treatment over prevention. It is estimated that there are currently 3 million people worldwide on antiviral cocktails. Yet for every two pursuing this treatment, there are five who are incubating the virus and are as yet undetected—a calculus of doom and failure. Prevention seems too bland, too simple. It lacks the "sizzle," the glamour and urgency of shining operating rooms and "wonder" drugs. We must also take into account the truth that, beyond the miseries and deaths caused by the preventable "big" conditions, they each involve huge treasuries of cash.

Another reason for our lack of a prevention strategy is fatalism. "You can't change human nature," is a remark that we hear much too often. The evidence to the contrary is critical. It is true that nature is intractable, but the medical contract involves more nurture than nature, and as such is eminently susceptible to choice and change.

Who "owns" prevention? Who is responsible for it? Earlier, I made the point that responsibility is a direct byproduct of knowledge. Benjamin Franklin asked, "How much responsibility does a newborn baby have?" The recent emphasis on information technology will provide our new design with the requisite "proof of concept" tools that the new paradigm demands.

Prevention is intrinsic to health. Until recently, we lacked knowledge of the biological mechanisms inherent in prevention. We had not defined the scientific principles, such as phenotypic plasticity, homeodynamics, and sym-morphosis, that describe health. In other words, we have not grasped how the organism and its environment work together to produce health and to protect against harm. Armed with an emerging new science of health, the arguments for prevention now take on rigor and substance. "Yes, we can," is a heraldic cry to new action.

Each of the following five medical conditions, which have enjoyed extensive investment of research and capital in repair techniques, is now susceptible to prevention by adopting the first principles of health.

## Preventing Heart Disease

It has been nearly 60 years since I wrote my honors thesis at Williams College on atherosclerosis, the underlying pathology of heart disease (5). These decades have generated hundreds of thousands of publications about the surgical and pharmaceutical approaches to this most common killer of the Western world. Someone facetiously commented that if medicine only had more stents (the sleeves that try to re-canalize blocked arteries) and statins (the class of drugs designed to lower blood cholesterol levels), we would be rid of this oppression. Such a suggestion defies reality. Half of heart attack deaths occur with the first attack, and treatment is clearly an ineffective option if you are dead.

Important in the debate about treatment versus prevention are what are termed risk factors, or early warning signals. There are risk factors for virtually every condition. Smoking is the obvious first example. Heart disease has its own list of risk factors, largely behavioral in nature and therefore correctable. Heart disease is a choice, not a fate, and addressing the risk factors is an obvious first-principles strategy.

We know the physical details of heart disease in great detail. The elucidation of the details of cholesterol formation earned a Nobel Prize. The mechanisms of blood clotting and arterial inflammatory response are extensively described in thousands of journal articles. These factors generate the two principal therapies of heart disease, surgery and drugs. Lacking in our pursuit of heart disease remediation is the grand adoption of a preventive strategy. We give it lip service, but we apply it inconsistently.

However, we have made some gains. Thirty years ago, the heart-related death statistics had been ominously worsening for decades. Then something happened: heart-related deaths began to drop—now they are 40% to 50% less than they were at their highest level. Experts debate the relative contribution of prevention versus treatment in this turnaround (6), but most acknowledge that both earlier aggressive treatment and improved behavioral patterns (lowered smoking levels are a major factor) played a role.

An important 2009 paper provided by medical professionals at the School of Medicine at the University of Minnesota and Health Partners Research Foundation in Minneapolis entitled "Comparative Effectiveness of Heart Disease Prevention and Treatment Strategies" constructs a model for "perfect care" in which all preventive goals were achieved by addressing risk factors, in addition to maximum drug and acute events therapy (7). The authors modeled a hypothetical cohort of 100,000 individuals 32 to 84 years of age and projected the number of deaths prevented or postponed (DPP) if "perfect care" intervention—prevention plus repair—was given to those of differing risks. For example, 90,000 of the 100,000 will have no heart disease, 8,300 will have heart disease without symptoms, and 1,600 will have known heart disease. Of the hundred thousand, 1,300 will die in 1 year of all causes, most of which would occur in the no-apparent-heart-disease group. Within 1 year, there would be 3,000 acute heart events, the most common scenario being out-of-the-hospital cardiac arrest.

The authors concluded that the largest increase in DPP from "perfect care" would result from increasing the physical activity of the asymptomatic group, followed by meeting dietary requirements and stopping smoking. Increasing physical activity was also the most powerful prevention strategy for those with known heart disease. One third of all deaths are prevented when perfect care is delivered to those with no known heart disease, while perfect care for all those known to have heart disease could prevent and postpone 23% of deaths.

This change in care would result in a 10- to 14-year increase in life expectancy. The authors comment that the reduction in heart disease risk factors also reduces the risk of death from other chronic diseases. "Conceptualizing heart disease as a chronic disease, rooted in behavior acquired early in life, rather than acute disease that strikes individuals in late life, is most likely to lead to breakthrough innovations," they write. Prevention trumps treatment.

Almost invisible in the background literature on heart disease is recognition of the size of the arteries. These tributaries are largely regarded as passive tubes to which bad things happen, clogging and inflammation among them.

Lacking in the general portrait is incorporation of the dynamic configuring of the artery to its inherent flow, its phenotypic plasticity. Recognizing that, according to Poiseuille's law, the flow to the tissues through the artery varies as the radius to the fourth power, the size issue is critical. Victor Dzau, now dean at Duke Medical School, has contributed several reports on the plasticity, or remodeling, of the vascular system, but most of his focus has been on the structural responses to various pathologic states (8).

There is great fascination with small or narrowed arteries, because they are precursors to interventional strategies. But we do not see a comparable interest in "big arteries," because they are not symptomatic—they are healthy. The work of Haskell and colleagues, published in *Circulation* in 1993, "Coronary Artery Size and Dilating Capacity in Ultradistance Runners," proved that the diameter of an artery responds to the flow within the artery, and the more flow, the larger the artery becomes in response (9). But I cannot find a category corresponding to "big arteries" in the medical literature. They get no recognition but are obviously of dominant significance in the story of heart disease. One can even ask, "Who cares what your cholesterol level is, if your artery is an inch across?" The prevention of heart disease should begin with a crusade for big arteries. The throb that accompanies a brisk walk or jog is the arteries stretching and reconfiguring to reflect greater flow.

A few years ago, our weekly grand rounds of the Department of Medicine here at Stanford (at which I am a never-fail attendee) featured a guest professor of notable credentials. His topic was angiogenesis. Angiogenesis, the formation of new blood vessels, is a hot frontier topic. The audience was breathless in anticipation. The speaker detailed the deep science underlying the process. He described how several key genes are inserted into a virus that nests in the targeted tissue to deliver the genes to the desired spot. Some time thereafter, there is evidence of new sproutings of small blood vessels. Considerable acclaim greeted this revelation. In the Q&A session, I asked, "But don't you get the same results from exercise?" He replied, "Of course. But there's no money in exercise."

## Preventing Cancer

The March 6, 2008, edition of the *New York Review of Books* features a cartoon in which the government is urging a medical scientist, "Could you please hurry and find a cure for cancer? That would be so much easier than prevention" (10). The cartoon references a review of *The Secret History of the War on Cancer* by Dr. Deborah Davis, director of the Center for Environmental Oncology at the

University of Pittsburgh Cancer Institute (11). Her main thesis is that the war on cancer has been fighting many of the wrong battles with the wrong weapons. The article itself cites the perspective of a British cancer scientist, Dr. Michael Sporin, who argues that the critical obstacle to large reductions in cancer mortality is a misplaced emphasis on treatment over prevention. Playing catch-up with surgery, radiation, and toxic drugs once cancer has taken hold reflects an inappropriate obsession with the concept of cure. In Sporin's words, "We must develop new approaches to control this plague of deaths by adopting an ethic of prevention, based on a more sophisticated understanding of the process of carcinogenesis and the potential to prevent disease before it becomes invasive and metastatic." Some call the present war on cancer futile. There has been no shortage in the nation's funding of cancer research, prompting one pundit to observe that "the more we spend the more we get." The return on investment is not impressive. The benefits have yet to justify the investment. It is notable that the great majority of the leaders in the cancer world, National Cancer Institute, American Cancer Society, and so on are of the repair fraternity—therapists. Radiation, surgery, and chemotherapy is their preoccupation.

Davis calls the accumulating evidence on environmental hazards a sign that these are perhaps *the* major preventable cause of malignant disease. Walter Willett, chief of the Harvard School of Public Health, estimates that 60% to 80% of cancers have an environmental cause (12). Among the many identified environmental factors are smoking, radiation, drugs, hormones, viruses, and organic solvents; surely there are others. The clustering of cancer cases in a particular environment is sometimes a clue.

Dr. Michael Marmot, professor of public health at the University of London, suggests that physical exercise, low-fat and low-sugar diets, and limiting one's consumption of meat, alcohol, and salt would prevent one third of all cancers—1.3 million new cases per year, 550,000 of whom will die (13). One half of males and one third of females will experience cancer in their lifetimes. But once again, contemporary medicine focuses on surgery and pills. Aside from a smattering of breakthrough therapies (see Lance Armstrong), cancer has not ceded its malevolence to surgery and pills. Next Medicine again acknowledges that cancer is partly caused by unidentified factors in the environment. Individual and collective responsibility calls for avoiding as many of those factors as possible: not smoking, using organic products, eating a diet rich in leafy vegetables, being careful about sun exposure, building lean muscle mass, and taking precautions against toxins at home and at work. It seems imperative that the National Cancer Institute and its attendant minions should embrace a new career of preventive oncology, using the language, equations, and metrics of Health Medicine.

## Preventing Diabetes

Diabetes was not a major part of my curriculum in medical school because it did not have much of a constituency. Fortunately, back in the 1950s, diabetes was still a rare disease. We studied only one kind; that was all that was recognized. Its current label is "type 1 diabetes, juvenile onset, insulin-dependent." Its cause is the destruction of the insulin-secreting cells of the pancreas due to a virus, which produces antibody products that maliciously attack and kill the beta cells. In my medical school days, we were excited to be provided with the first crude tools of insulin, the result of Banting and Best's historic discovery in 1922. This new treatment allowed diabetics to live, whereas previously their death warrant had been sealed. However, the quality of the lives extended was diminished by the awful complications of blindness, kidney failure, and more.

An article in the *Annals of Internal Medicine* in November 1924 by Herman Emerson and Louise Carson of the Public Health School of Columbia was called "Diabetes Mellitus, a Contribution to Its Epidemiology Based Chiefly on Mortality Statistics" (14). This paper was a rendering of the causes of death for the city of New York for the years 1866 to 1922, the year when insulin was born. In 1866, there were 11 deaths recorded from diabetes out of a population of 770,000; four of these patients were under 25 years of age and five were over 45. In 1923, there were 1,360 deaths of diabetes in a population of 5.4 million, 54 of whom were under 20 years of age, 1,213 over 45. The rate of death from diabetes of 2 per 100,000 in 1866 rose to 22 per 100,000 in 1922. The death rates from diabetes were negligible for laborers, but 180 per hundred thousand for bartenders and 120 per hundred thousand for clergymen, the next highest category. In the years since these statistics were collected, the world has become older and more diabetic. The current estimate of the number of people with diabetes in America is 23 million (15). The CDC projects that one third of the children born this year will become diabetic; for Hispanic and African-American babies, that number rises to a staggering 50%. There are 800,000 new cases reported per year and 200,000 associated deaths. The Yale School of Public Health recently reported that these numbers may triple by 2030 (16).

There is a defined condition called prediabetes in which the blood sugar is elevated but not yet to the level required to make the diagnosis official (17). There are millions of these waiting in the wings. Beyond this category, I have previously coined a new term, pre-prediabetes, to classify those hundred million other overfed and underfit persons whose blood sugar levels have not yet started to climb as they spend down their precious reserves (18). It seems likely that diabetes in one way or another affects every single person in the United States. However, startling as all these statistics are, they probably represent underestimates because of the documented underreporting of this often-silent disease.

Even armed with much new knowledge about diabetes and potential treatments, the therapeutic results are very imperfect. Diabetes results in an average life shortening of 15 years, and 15 years times 20 million people equals an unconscionable amount of life lost. Perhaps worse, diabetes is cruel in the miseries that it causes before it kills: it is the number-one cause of blindness, the number-one cause of kidney failure, and the number-one cause of peripheral vascular disease and amputation.

Type 1 diabetes, the end result of an immune-mediated destruction of the islet cells of the pancreas, putatively attributed to a virus, remains a significant health threat, but the categorically different disease of type 2 diabetes, maturity-onset diabetes, is where the real problem resides. I have differentiated types 1 and 2 with automobile analogies. In the first instance, it is a car with a hole in the gas tank, which requires a constant external supply of insulin. In type 2 the car has enough gas but is pulling a trailer full of tons of cinder blocks, wearing everything out. Providing more insulin in the second case is of secondary concern. Fifty years ago we did not even recognize or identify type 2 because it was so rare. There were some older people with elevated blood sugar levels, but we attributed these levels to age rather than a certified disease. However, type 2 really is not maturity-onset, because pediatricians are seeing thousands of children with it.

Intimate to any discussion of the pathologies of diabetes are the costs that accompany them. The American Diabetes Association (ADA) conservatively puts the cost of diabetes currently at $180 billion per year, or 7% of the GDP (15). Perhaps one in five of all health care dollars are consumed, directly or indirectly, by diabetes. Further, the ADA points out that costs per person with the disease are $15,000 per year, or $11,000 above the non-diabetic cost of $4,000 per person per year. Multiply this $15,000 times 20 million, and you derive huge dollar amounts that become paralyzing in what they portend.

The drug industry has developed and promoted dozens of new drugs to assist overworked doctors who have patients with type 2 diabetes, but these are only a feeble effort, and an inappropriate approach. So once again, Current Medicine reaches into its little black bag and extracts surgery for weight loss and diabetes control, officially known as bariatric, obesity, or weight-loss surgery. Stomach bypass centers advertise on everything from highway billboards to little-traveled Web sites—this has been likened to a Wild West free-for-all with plenty of guns for hire. The April 25, 2008, issue of *Science* magazine contains a major article, "Bypassing Medicine to Treat Diabetes," that describes the new rage (19). Back in the 1950s, stomach surgery for cancer and ulcers was accompanied by weight loss and reduced blood sugar levels, but not until recently was it proposed to use these side effects as a treatment for diabetes. It is estimated that 200,000 of these procedures were performed in 2008 (20). I am disheartened that even my academic home of Stanford has brought on a bariatric surgeon to exploit this bonanza. But a consideration of the numbers involved indicates that we will need to train tens of thousands of bariatric surgeons if they hope to keep up with the demand. I am profoundly embarrassed that my profession insists that major surgery is an appropriate therapy for a behavioral condition; we may as well recommend finger amputation to prevent smoking.

As compelling as all the numbers relating to the categorical disease called diabetes are, they are marginalized by the fact that diabetes is in reality much more than diabetes, a pathology principally characterized as a disorder of carbohydrate metabolism. It has long been known that persons with diabetes rarely die from diabetes *per se*; more commonly they die of associated cardiovascular disease. The hallmarks of heart disease are elevated blood fat levels, high blood pressure, and the rest of the risk factors for circulatory problems.

High levels of sugar in the blood are often associated with lipid abnormalities. In fact, this combination of findings—elevated blood sugar, elevated cholesterol levels, and high blood pressure—was found so consistently together that they have been melded into another single diagnosis called the "metabolic syndrome." This term has gained popularity because it enlarges the notion of diabetes as a deficit in carbohydrate metabolism to reflect a more generalized set of problems. The category of metabolic syndrome grew rapidly until it was challenged by cardiologists, who felt that the term underrecognized the strong presentation of circulatory problems in those with this condition. They proposed a new term, "cardiometabolic syndrome" or "metabo-cardiac syndrome." The turf war continues, with different interest groups of competing specialties loath to relinquish bragging and naming rights.

I have been an interested observer of this drama because it reflects directly on Current Medicine's insistence on reductionistic messaging. The heart doctors and the gland doctors each claim primacy of billing for what is eventually a system condition, describable and included in the earlier formulations of the disuse syndrome, hypokinetic disease, exercise deficiency disorder, or sedentary death syndrome (21–23). All of these groupings include diabetes. But the diabetes component is only a fraction of the bigger picture. Next Medicine has much work to do in its insistence on a "systems" approach and taxonomy.

The twin therapies of Current Medicine, surgery and pills, are fully employed in treating diabetes and its related syndromes. But a moment's reflection reveals that the actual diagnosis, the actual cause, is not susceptible to pills or surgery, but is largely preventable if the patient makes a simple, safe, cheap, and effective lifestyle adjustment. The central counterpoint to the ineffective therapies that are being put forth by contemporary medicine for diabetes is the multicenter trial called the Diabetes Prevention Project. This crucial experiment conducted at nine centers across the country was led by David Nathan of Boston, and the results were published in the *New England Journal of Medicine* in 2002 (24). It showed that a very modest lifestyle modification, adding physical exercise and nutritional counseling, was able to prevent onset of the disease in 58% of a large group of prediabetic persons who were otherwise destined to develop it shortly.

## Preventing Arthritis

My favorite medical index Web site, PubMed of the National Library of Medicine, reveals 7,346 articles on the prevention of arthritis, but 94,719 on its treatment. The index term "prevention of osteoarthritis," the most common form of arthritis, reveals 1,671 citations, but there are 23,446 citations on osteoarthritis treatment. I was surprised that the preventive category would show up at all, because virtually nobody mentions the prevention of arthritis in professional discussions.

I have long maintained that movement and high quality of life are tightly linked. Earlier I proposed that our species' survival was utterly dependent on mobility. This linkage is apparent at all stages of life but becomes increasingly evident as the decades pass. The most common diagnosis among older people is arthritis. There are various estimates of its incidence, but in very old people, it is likely that all will show some sign of it.

First, a little background. Osteoarthritis is the result of biomechanical injury. The lining surface of all joints is cartilage, vertically oriented molecules of mucopolysaccharide and chondroitin sulfate. The healthy joint displays an orderly orientation of these molecules that is wonderfully maintained by the appropriate compressive forces being applied across the joint (think Golden Mean again) (25). Too much or too little mechanical force, misalignment, or torsion leads to disruption of that order. Our joints, like the rest of our anatomical equipment, possess a substantial energetic margin before injury becomes apparent. There is often a long lag between initial injury or continued overuse before evidence of arthritis appears, compounding the challenges of analysis. The joint's subsequent efforts to repair itself lead to the knobby appearance that is the visible evidence of healing. In 1983, Dr. John Bland, one of our most respected authorities on arthritis, published a paper in the *American Journal of Medicine* titled "The Reversibility of Arthritis," in which he showed X-ray pictures of improvement in the arthritic change after the aberrant mechanical forces were realigned (26). Certain mechanical features, such as obesity, bow-legs, and knock-knees, predispose to osteoarthritis, as does being a professional football lineman, or a ballerina, or a rodeo rider. As noted previously, an NIH study revealed that leg strength was the single best predictor of the need for nursing home placement in late life.

So I wonder why we have not developed a specialty of preventive orthope-dics. Some of my best friends are therapeutic orthopedists, and my family has benefited greatly from their competence. But what about the prevention of arthritis in the first place? Since osteoarthritis is the end result of decades of inappropriate molecular forces at the joint surface, I advocate for the preventive orthopedist to periodically generate a skeletal survey, a Cybex machine-like assessment in which the various vectors, angles, and forces of the joint spaces are mapped and any laxity or tightness is identified. Then early corrective efforts could be undertaken in muscle strength and laxity to restore the joint to its proper symmetry, all to prevent arthritis. Now, the pharmaceutical firms that provide us with tons of arthritis medicines and the manufacturers of the ware-houses full of replacement joints will not rise in support of an arthritis preven-tion protocol, despite the fact that their knees and backs will be relieved not to have to support the heavy wallets that bulge with the profits from arthritis treatment.

Osteoporosis is a kindred skeletal disease for which under-loading of the skeleton is a substantial contribution, again a situation that begs for a preven-tive strategy. The National Osteoporosis Foundation Web site begins with a statement that preventing osteoporosis is important because there is no cure, and prevention is readily attainable: engage in weight-bearing exercise, get optimal amounts of calcium and vitamin D, avoid smoking and excessive alcohol consumption, and so on (27).

## Preventing Brain Diseases

As we age, a principal specter in the list of health threats is the category of neurologic disorders such as strokes, Alzheimer's disease, and Parkinson's disease. The online editorial in the *Annals of Neurology* on June 3, 2009, by workers from the Karolinska Institute in Stockholm, was entitled "Preventive Neurology" (28). Rather than accepting the traditional passive clinical posture to these pathologies, the article recognizes a new approach that urges a switch to an aggressive prevention stance. A corollary review article by workers from the Memory and Brain Health Center in Baltimore calls the new perspective "the dynamic polygon hypothesis." Instead of brain disorders being held to be the reductionistic simplistic sequence of single process/single outcome, now proposed is the notion that these deteriorations exist with multiple causes and multiple approaches, including the powerful implication of lifestyle issues, a "system" rather than a "component" heuristic (29).

Such a major revision in conceptual framework emphasizes preventive strategies. Workers at the University of Washington in Seattle reported on the effects of aerobic exercise in individuals with mild cognitive impairment in the January 2010 issue of the *Archives of Neurology* (30). In 33 subjects 6 months of aerobic training resulted in "significant gains in mental agility when contrasted with controls, who exhibited continued decline." Major new scientific discoveries emerge about the physiologic mechanisms responsible for these findings, such as the elevation in brain-derived neurotrophic factor (BDNF) with exercise (31).

Each of these conditions screams for a comprehensive prevention strategy. Larry Cohen of the Prevention Institute in Oakland has put together a useful guide, *Prevention Is Primary*, which suggests a hierarchical approach to constructing a "culture of prevention". Its steps are (1) strengthening individual knowledge and skills, (2) promoting community education, (3) educating providers, (4) fostering coalitions and networks, (5) changing organizational practices, and (6) influencing policy and legislation (32).

As Next Medicine establishes the template for prevention strategies, it needs a generic planning process for the multilevel approaches that will be involved. Next Medicine dictates that we commit to making these strategies a higher priority than they are now, with expanded investment in personnel, technology, and dollars.

It is the replacement paradigm. Higher taxes will not fix Americans' health, nor will politically driven health care reform. Increased debt won't do it either. Prevention will.

# Healthier Living and Aging: *Mens* | 10
## *Sana in Corpore Sano*

Some years ago I arranged a seminar at the Center for Advanced Study in the Behavioral Sciences at Stanford University. I did this to cement my new friendship with Norman Cousins, whom I had originally contacted about his memorable article in the *New England Journal of Medicine,* "Anatomy of an Illness" (1). This autobiographical case report recorded his experience with a severe rheumatoid syndrome at a top New York hospital. Cousins' take on this experience was that he was steadily deteriorating as parts of him were being taken off to assorted laboratories by anonymous scientists who never saw him as a person, but only as an object of scientific curiosity. Famously, Cousins injected laughter into his cure. *Candid Camera* and Groucho Marx were his therapists. He got better.

I was so taken by his story that I invited him to share a panel with me at an AMA meeting on wellness in Las Vegas. Linus Pauling, who knew Cousins from their World Federalist Association encounters, happened to be in the front row of our session. Cousins and I hit it off famously. I considered it a privileged role to constrain his enthusiastic embrace of mental attitude in all health encounters: "You are right Norman, but...." It was in this spirit that I arranged the Stanford seminar. Also invited were assorted neuroscientists, including Tom Gonda, chairman of psychiatry at Stanford; Seymour Kety of Harvard; and the granddaddy of the theory of the chemical basis of schizophrenia,

Jack Barcus, now professor of psychiatry at Cornell and then head of the neurotransmitter lab. He and I and several others had collaborated on a *New England Journal of Medicine* article on endorphins and exercise (2).

We surrounded a conference table for several hours as the assembled scientists detailed their work on the esoterica of depression, affect disorders, and schizophrenia. Cousins sat silent until right before lunch. He then calmly said, "We have spent three hours hearing of the malfunctions of these brain disorders. Fascinating stuff, but is there not a complementary position, a healthy brain? A healthy biology aspect in contrast to the disease biology? What about hope and altruism and love? Do not these mental constructs also affect how the brain works?" Our group was stunned for a moment, but quickly concurred that the healthy emotions were certainly secreted from the brain in a way similar to the psychoses and neuroses. We all recognized the method in Cousins' query. Subsequently, he went on to help fund the Psychoimmunology Department at the UCLA School of Medicine, which validated what he thought about the effect that healthy emotions have on the body.

## Mens Sana

*Mens sana in corpore sano*, a healthy mind in a healthy body, has echoed through history—starting with the Roman poet Juvenal, who coined the phrase as part of an answer to what we should want in life (3). Over time, it has had a range of meanings, from "only a healthy body can produce a healthy mind," to the opposite, the need for a balance of health in both mind and body.

But only recently have the structure and function of the healthy brain been known in any detail. For almost the entire period of our existence until this time, the brain has been interpreted largely by mystics and hypnotists. Freud *et al.* proved to be of little explanatory help in the real world. The 1990s became known as the decade of the brain because of the extraordinary advancements in neuroscience. The wonderful new imaging techniques, together with an explosive increase in our knowledge of brain chemistry, have provided insights into ephemeral domains such as consciousness and memory. Such competence in the medical world comes at just the right time because of the new upsurge in our older population, which brings with it a novel set of neurological disorders, including Alzheimer's and Parkinson's disease, which distort the image of healthy aging. Who would choose to be old and mindless at the same time? We need broad enlightenment. The biology and psychology of life become increasingly relevant as we age. Mental competence has a timeline, but like the body, the brain is wonderfully trainable. I often think of the brain, whose structure and function balance precisely, in "use it or lose it" terms. The brain is much like a muscle.

Peter Laslett was a distinguished British historian and gerontologist. He had an abiding commitment to expanding our ideas about aging, and urged rejection of many of the stereotypes. In pursuit of this ideal he started the University of the Third Age in Cambridge in 1981 (4). He said, "The greatest part of the human life potential has been wasted by people who die before their allotted time is up."

Newly helping us to define the "last of life for which the first is made" is a broad-based international research effort to aggregate for purposes of study the "supercentenarians," those persons who are now credentialed as being over 110 years old. A paper by Schoenhofen and colleagues from the University of Southern California in the 2006 *Journal of American Geriatrics Society*, "Characteristics of 32 Supercentenarians," concluded that "a surprisingly substantial proportion of these individuals were still functionally independent or required minimal assistance" (5).

Globally, several research groups are eagerly searching out diverse populations where supercentenarianism seems to be the norm. These areas include Sardinia, Japan, Okinawa, Costa Rica, Greece, and the Seventh-Day Adventist Church in Loma Linda, California. Collectively, they are known as the "blue zone" (6). A 2009 expedition to Ikaria in Greece uncovered the highest percentage of 90-year-olds on the planet. Nearly one in three people there make it into their nineties. They have much less cancer and heart disease and almost no dementia (7). The workers are receiving support from the National Geographic Society, which seems to maintain a commitment in getting this story out. Recall that 30 years ago there was a published similar effort on three populations in southern Russia, Hunza (Pakistan), and Ecuador (8). Unfortunately, scholar-sleuths determined that the featured subjects had fraudulently inflated their ages, so the current investigators are being meticulous in their characterization.

Surveying these groups for commonalities the researchers, find (1) constant moderate physical activity, which seems to be an inseparable part of their life; (2) no smoking; (3) a plant-based diet; and (4) social engagement, with close contact and devotion to family and community.

Establishing a blue zone at this date encourages us to seek strategies that will enlarge the number included in fulfilling a life potential. Conversely, one might investigate the red zone, those parts of the world where longevity is foreshortened, and see what the common characteristics are. I would guess they would include physical inactivity, a high-fat and sugar-rich diet, smoking, and a high incidence of social disengagement. Does this sound familiar? No wonder our international health ranking is so poor and may be sinking further (9).


## Engagement and Flow

One of the key behavioral strategies in a successful life is engagement. Men and women are social creatures. People need people. This interdependency is evidenced in innumerable studies that show how social isolation is not good for you. Loneliness is a killer. One of the expressions of our social dependency goes by the term "engagement." Behavioral scientists measure engagement the way I measure blood pressure. Engagement is quantified by the number of interactive encounters a person experiences in a given period of time. Interactions reflect the body encountering its environment. The numbers of phone calls, letters written, sexual experiences, clubs joined, newspapers read—each encounter is a specific individual response.

When Elaine Cumming and William Henry of the University of Chicago assessed engagement events over the course of a lifetime in their 1961 book *Growing Old*, they plotted a declining slope with a steeper tilt toward the end (10). Is this disengagement an inevitable result of aging or, as Stanford's Laura Carstensen surmised, something else? She measured the engagement quotient of a group of gay people, and found that these subjects were at least as engaged as the straight community (11). However, when they transited to an HIV-positive state, their engagement numbers tilted downward; when they became ill with AIDS, they shriveled and withdrew. Her conclusion is that disengagement for many people is not aging *per se*, but a covert anticipation of dying, a gradual relinquishing of life.

A haunting subsequent question arises: What if it is not time yet? What if this often-depressed person is not aware that the natural health span is, as I posit, 100 years? The analogy of behavioral disengagement with the receptor site and the engagement of the soma involve the interreactivity of the mind and body with the environment. As I have said, disengagement disrupts energy flow, which is essential for both mental and physical health. This newly elaborated feature of healthy psychological being describes the qualitative nature of daily experience. Mihaly Czikszentmihalyi of the Claremont Graduate University codified this process with the word "flow" (12). Flow describes phenomena that are effortless, timeless, unforced, automatic, and usually pure pleasure. Like the other parameters above, we take flow for granted. Czikszentmihalyi does not: he measures it. For this he uses the experience sampling method. He asks that the study subject carry a beeper in his or her pocket. This beeper goes off irregularly and the subject is asked to record the time, the perceived level of flow, and what is going on at the moment. After Czikszentmihalyi aggregated thousands of records of all ages, ethnicities, incomes, genders, the processes of who has flow, how much, and when, the straightforward results read as follows: Flow occurs optimally when the person is engaged in a task that is challenging and rewarding. Flow does not occur at a time of idleness or purely hedonistic pursuit, and it notably does not occur while watching television. If, on the other hand, the task is greater than the person's perceived ability to accomplish it (self-efficacy), then stress results. When a task is less challenging than the capacity available for the test, then boredom ensues. Flow occurs at the idealized intersection of capacity and task, of organism and environment (Fig. 10.1). All of which harks back to Aristotle, and the notion of the Golden Mean.

In 2003, Frank Hu of the Harvard School of Public Health surveyed people's brain metabolism while they watched TV and found that their brain oxygen consumption was equal to that when regarding a brick wall (13). It was on a par with stupor, with energy flow at a virtual standstill. Thus the psychological profile of health engagement and flow conforms precisely with the parameters inherent in physical health. *Mens sana in corpore sano;* all is harmony.

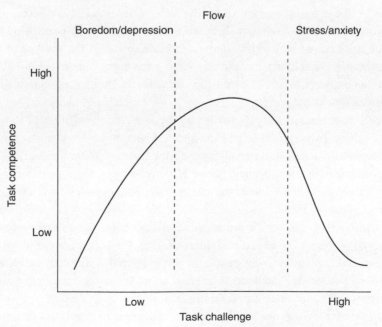

**Figure 10.1** Flow.

## Healthier Aging

Because of the many events and shaping forces that surround us as we age, our trajectories vary. Tom Perls categorizes three of these trajectories: "escapers," "survivors," and "endurers" (14). The escaper is the lucky person who arrives at an advanced age without having had a substantial encounter with a debilitating, destabilizing event. The survivor is the individual who has had one or more adverse encounters in life but has managed by skill, resolve, nature, or luck to live to fight another day. The endurer is the plucky or unfortunate person who has not drawn the lucky hand but still has managed to stay the course. It is likely that most people have elements of each of these trajectories in their life stories.

Another way to think about aging: eminent gerontologists Jack Rowe and Robert Kahn wrote an influential article in *Science* in 1987 in which they differentiated between usual aging and successful aging (15). To me, "usual aging" implies a disease-free aging, but one that still contains the multiple decremental signs of disuse. "Successful aging" connotes the ideally functioning individual with all systems go. For example, studies on patients in nursing homes revealed the real-life lesson that derives from urging the residents to retain their vigor and maintain their environments. The challenged residents live longer and have many fewer hospital visits. Even older patients in the ICU do as well as younger patients if their functional state is considered.

Until the past few years, the entire field of aging was a wasteland. It was informed largely by demographers who preached the perils of growing older. Geriatrics lacked a historical context. It has also lacked the prestige of other domains. Until recently, the science of aging has been a muddle of mislabeling and ignorance. Current Medicine has clumsily tried to fit aging into its disease format. It does not fit.

The population change predicted by the Age Wave (two thirds of all people in the world who have reached the age of 65 are now alive) caused tremors. Margaret Thatcher, when challenged about Britain's grand strategy for confronting the age boom, replied, "I hear that is coming. I just hope it does not hit on my watch." America hears the alarm, but other countries are in even worse shape. Former Secretary of Commerce Peter G. Peterson's book *Gray Dawn* calculates that the world's unfunded social program commitments (entitlements) represent the $64 trillion question (16). He cites a current $35 trillion unfunded liability for older people in the industrial world. Italy has it worst, suffering from the "Bambino Bust" and about to become the first nation in history with more citizens over 60 than under 20.

America, by contrast, is relatively young, the result largely of our generous immigration policies. Still, 4 million Americans turn 65 every year. The Social

Security Administration (SSA) provides much entertainment in its theoretical projections of future age trends. One scenario using a hypothetical decrease of 2% per year for mortality would lead to an average population longevity of 104 in 2030 and 115 by 2075 (17). The *Lancet* October 2009 issue projects that half of the children in the developed world born since 2000 can expect to become centenarians (18). It is certain that this realization will not occur because of the contents of a pill bottle. Jane Brody's *New York Times* column of January 11, 2010, is titled "Healthy Aging, with Nary a Supplement" (19). The SSA notes that for recent history, Japanese mortality has fallen even faster, at 5% per year.

Japan and China face huge aging challenges (20). Since the beginning of our species, children have been the old-age insurance that represented sturdy bulwarks of family support. With the population-limiting policies in China and Japan, a rapid redistribution of their age cohorts looms. Japan, famous for its custom of older people living with their children, now needs nursing homes. The Chinese face an unimaginable prospect of having 330 million citizens over 65 in 2050. The country faces a chilling future with a sparse cohort of female youngsters due to their one-child-per-family policy. Worldwide, the family tree is growing taller and older but slimmer, with fewer branches.

Policy planners and sociologists are asking two critical questions: Will the world's nations grow rich or old first? Will our aging selves be a resource or a liability? Stanford economist John Shoven notes that aging inevitably distorts fiscal projections. There is a large possibility that society is confronting a fiscal train wreck. One optimistic suggestion is that old people represent our only natural resource that is increasing. This possibility exists, but it has no warranty. Pete Peterson comments that working longer is not *an* answer to the financial worries (16), it is *the* answer. But working longer, as desirable a strategy as it is, deeply depends on vitality, vigor, and fitness. If our millions of older selves enter later age feeble and dependent, then disaster looms.

In 1982, I wrote in *JAMA*: "There is no drug in current or prospective use that holds nearly so much hope for a full vital life as one lived with physical exercise" (21). This sentiment lay fallow for more than 20 years, until I was roused by the introduction of the Medicare Drug Entitlement Bill. This legislation is destined to cost future taxpayers trillions of dollars, and the principal beneficiaries will be the stockholders of Merck, Pfizer, and the other drug companies. I was activated sufficiently to call Senator Dianne Feinstein's office and make my case. I was then referred to Florida Senator Robert Graham's office, since he was the prime mover of this legislation. Soon I was on the phone to a staffer, who allowed me to rant briefly before interrupting and telling me, "Stop, of course you are right. People need to take a walk instead of a pill, but we are in receipt of 30 million e-mails from members of the AARP, who are anxious for the bill to ride through. We are beholden to this message." I was upset by this fatalistic political reality, but then he said, "What do you want us to do?" His comprehension of the inadequacy of a pharmaceutical approach to healthy aging has been echoed by a number of government health authorities, and I am optimistic that the opportunity now presents itself to address what the drug bill addressed inappropriately.

How much of the bad rap that aging has accumulated is time-coded? Satchel Paige's challenge, "How old would you be if you didn't know how old you were?" throws the spotlight on attitude. I have often written that "aging is a self-fulfilling prophecy" and constantly make the point that we are largely liable for our own destiny. We set our course, not fate. In *Walking Naked,* British novelist Nina Bawden warns us not to succumb to the fear, not of death, but of all the indignities lying in wait for us (22). In *Human Options,* Norman Cousins wrote, "Nothing about life is more precious than that we can define our own destinies" (23). The crowning advice on aging may also come from Cousins: "Any life, however long, is too short if it is bereft of splendor, the passions under-worked, the memories sparse and the imagination unlit by radiant musing."

## Parkinson's and Alzheimer's

Two biological conditions pervade our older years: neurological disorders and frailty. Parkinson's disease and Alzheimer's disease are co-conspirators. I learned virtually nothing about these conditions when I was in medical school. They were known, but they had only a small constituency. But with the rapid crush in the number of older people, these diseases have become commonplace and familiar. Much of the image of aging is shrouded by the ugly specters of Alzheimer's and Parkinson's disease.

Parkinsonism starts predominantly as a motor deficit, with rigidity and tremor as prime symptoms. Alzheimer's disease starts as a falter in cognitive capacity affecting mostly recent memory. As the years drag slowly on, the two conditions turn the patient into a pathetic caricature of his or her former self. The diseases are especially malevolent in the burden they put on family caregivers, who usually hurt more than those actually affected by the disease. Unfortunately, the medical system has no satisfactory remedies for either in its little black bag. Millions of lives are distorted by these diseases.

The search for a specific cause of both has not succeeded, but there is early indication that a breakthrough may be near. Borrowing on insights provided by other neurological diseases such as epilepsy, a novel pathogenic mechanism suggests that the targeted brain cells of Alzheimer's and Parkinsonism simply starve to death because of the loss of the predominant biochemical machinery that is responsible for combusting carbohydrates—converting sugar to energy. Oddly, the cells retain their capacity to burn ketone bodies derived from fat metabolism for energy, and when this alternative foodstuff is supplied, the cells spruce up and the symptoms improve.

Despite earlier fatalism concerning these conditions, I am currently hopeful, specifically because of the work of colleagues like Bud Veech at the NIH and Kieran Clarke at Oxford (24). Together they are pursuing a totally different nutritional path to these diseases, and if early results hold up, we may be truly headed for a gilded age in which much of the fear of these conditions would be erased. If the results are sustained and these awful conditions are scrubbed off our list of debilities of the aged, then we will be thoroughly charged to attack the more generic and more systemic condition of frailty.

## Frailty

Frailty is the number-one pathology of old people. It dominates our concept of "old." But frailty is not equivalent to aging. My interest in it goes back to a clumsy episode on the Nose Dive ski run at Stowe, Vermont. This embarrassment left me with my right leg in a cast for 6 weeks following a surgical repair of my torn Achilles tendon. I was astonished when the cast was removed and I saw a precociously frail leg. How had it become so old and frail? The other leg was just as old and it was fine. The fact was that if the surgeon had put the cast on the good leg, it would have suffered the same change. My leg became rapidly frail because it was immobile for so long.

Many older people are vigorous, and some young people are frail. The idea that frailty has something to do with aging is inescapable, though, because it so frequently accompanies age. Although it has a time dimension, it is not the same as aging. Frailty is reversible. And it is not an acute condition. Neither is it a disease. In medical school I had no courses on frailty. It is not included as a topic in many geriatrics texts. Frailty, like aging, has lacked a definition. I could not admit a patient to the hospital with a diagnosis of frailty. Similarly, it is not sanctioned on a death certificate. Like McGinnis and Foege's "Actual Causes of Death," frailty may be "a" or "the" major cause of death (25). Much has been written about the inaccuracy of the recorded causes of death on death certificates. I can certainly testify that I was complicit in this. In filling out death certificates for hundreds of patients whose cause of death was obscure, I typically wrote down "cardiac arrest as a result of arteriosclerosis," when I probably should have written "frailty." The most common pathology, catabolism of older persons, is frailty, but it is not a categorical disease. So what is it?

Nowadays, largely thanks to the explanation provided by thermodynamics, we have a tangible framework we can act on the basis of. Frailty is a system-wide state with function that has been reduced to less than 30% of normal, which involves the total organism, which is therefore prone to failure. Linda Fried's (who is now at Columbia) group at the Johns Hopkins Center on Aging and Health has done the most to define frailty (26). She calls frailty a syndrome, a cycle in which musculoskeletal, neuroendocrine, nutritional, and immuno-logical defects are present. Her group has enlarged our body of knowledge on the causes and remedies of frailty, finding that exercise is the basis of successful intermediation. My own work has built on her pioneering efforts (27).

Because frailty, unlike aging, is to a large extent reversible and preventable, the stakes are high. Acknowledging this, I contend that the common gateway condition that leads to frailty is muscular weakness, the result of protracted disuse. Data from the Framingham study, ongoing since 1948, reveal that 30% of women over 65 cannot walk 800 yards (28). In his last book, *Going the Distance*, my running friend George Sheehan wrote, "Age is the combat for which I'm training" (29). All of this has led me to champion the idea that the legs, not the brain, or the heart, or the lungs, are the most important organ in the older person's body. The fittest survive a lesson first taught millions of years ago on the Serengeti and endorsed today. I have often argued that the trajectory of late life is largely a choice, not fate. Employing the definitions, language, and metrics of Health Medicine, Next Medicine must arm us with the required medical framework to confront the epidemic of frailty in an enlightened and hopeful way.

We cannot "cure" aging, but we can relieve its burdens.

## Aging and Sexuality

Since sex is a major quality-of-life issue for most people, regardless of age, and since medicine's mission is to ensure human potential, it follows that robust sexuality with aging is a top agenda item for Next Medicine. Not surprisingly, sexuality increasingly emerges as a significant life-potential feature.

When I lecture on successful aging, I often encounter the question of why women outlive men. We do not have the answer to that yet, but I argue that the prime determinants of self-efficacy for the aging male are job and sexuality. The two epaulets on the male uniform are career satisfaction and sexual satisfaction. When these two prime identifying emblems are removed, the man stands naked

and vulnerable. Just days before his suicide, Ernest Hemingway spoke despair-
ingly of the state of his life: "What does a man care about? Staying healthy.
Working good. Eating and drinking with his friends. Enjoying himself in bed.
I haven't any of them. Do you understand, goddamn it? None of them!" (30)
Tragically, this scenario occurs frequently.

Since I recognized the importance of sex in late life, I have labored to
become better informed on this topic, which has been a long-standing Victorian
taboo for medicine. Alfred Kinsey, followed a generation later by William
Masters and Virginia Johnson, had much to do with leading us out of the darkness
on this topic (31,32). Alex Comfort's *The Joy of Sex* titillated and informed (33).
To educate myself, I have done research and written three papers on the subject.
In 2007, "A Study of Sexuality and Health Among Older Adults in the United
States" was published in the *New England Journal of Medicine* by a study team
from the University of Chicago and the University of Toronto (34). Their cohort
of 3,005 older adults (1,550 females and 1,455 males), 57 to 85 years of age, was
given an extensive questionnaire. Their results confirmed those of my earlier
research and others. First, older people are more sexually active than generally
recognized. Even the 75- to 85-year-olds reported having sex two or three times
per month, and 23% claimed a frequency of once a week or more; 87% of the
older men claimed that sex was still important to them. Good news.

But both men and women reported problems: 37% of the males reported
impotency, and 14% were actually taking medications to improve their erectile
function. All reports indicate that the male problem of impotency was highly
correlated with overall health status, medication use, and lack of an actively
participating mate. The issues for older women are somewhat different. Their
most cited lament is lack of a male partner. Erica Jong, Betty Friedan, and
Bonnie Matheson have written passionately on this issue (35–37). There is currently a surge in interest by the pharmaceutical world in the most common
syndrome of older women, hypoactive female desire syndrome. Their drugs
target centers in the brain that control the erotic appetite, to stimulate them in
older women. I await the research papers. Where can I invest?

We men must do a better job of surviving. An article in the February 2008
issue of the *Archives of Internal Medicine* by Dr. Laurel Yates and colleagues
from the Divisions of Aging and Preventive Medicine at Harvard was titled
"Exceptional Longevity in Men" (38). They followed 2,357 healthy males of the
Physicians' Health Study, with an average age of 72, for 16 years. Of this group,
970, or 41%, survived at least until age 90. 54% of those who did not smoke and
were not diabetic, overweight, hypertensive, or sedentary lived to age 90. Not
only did these habits favor survival, but better health and function persisted,
keeping many women happy.

In 1997, an article in the *British Medical Journal* asked, "Sex and Death; Are They Related?" (39) The authors surveyed 1,222 men aged 45 to 57, the entire male population of Caerphilly, South Wales, with 918 completing the sexuality part of the questionnaire. Ten years of follow-up revealed that the sexually active men had half the mortality of the inactive group. And furthermore, the protection was dose-dependent—in other words, the more sex, the greater the life extension. An accompanying editorial to the Wales study, also in the *BMJ,* was titled, "Just What the Doctor Ordered, More Alcohol and Sex." Underscoring the problem inherent in these surprising discoveries, the author writes, "What we thought was bad for you may actually be good for you, but it may not be good to tell you in case you do it too much. It is certainly not good to tell you it is good for you if you do too much of it already" (40).

Next Medicine requires a well-tuned antenna for further evidence of improvement strategies for late-life sexuality in both sexes. We need all the help that Next Medicine and its new signaling can bring to the agenda. With the world's population growing older, it is imperative that Medicine establish a comprehensive plan to confront it, realistically and effectively. Despite the lures of the mythical fountain of youth, aging cannot be cured. But when aging is armed with self-efficacy and engagement, it fills out the last of life with vitality and function. Once again, it is not how old you are that matters, but how you are old.

# Closing the Loop: Healthy Death | 11

An unexpected dividend of pursuing a career in geriatric medicine is that it brings a greater experience in and familiarity with death and dying. Accepting the role of caring steward of life's end casts the geriatrician in the role of staring one's patient's death squarely in the eye and gradually learning not to blink. One's learning provides no guidance for fulfilling this precious role. The medical school curriculum offers no instruction sheet on dying; internship and residency are likewise blank slates when it comes to teaching young doctors how to preside at this delicate time. Doctors are almost universally unfamiliar with death and are usually awkward and unsure of the script. Groucho Marx's comic persona Dr. Quackenbush's remark, "Either this man is dead or my watch has stopped" is a rude, if not entirely inaccurate, description of this general ineptitude.

But beyond the physician's discomfort in helping the ultimate curtain drop lies the possibility of making things worse than they already are. Many years ago I sketched out the additional challenges the physician confronts when choosing a career with older people as clientele. The first arises from the recognition that very few of us live as long as I argue that our owner's manual says that we can, and the physician is constantly struggling to assess how best to assure the patient of his or her allotted lifetime.

The second challenge is equally unsettling. Our new technological competence arms the physician with tools of formidable power, the ability to sustain a low level of life far longer than the warranty is intended to last. Nothing is worse than the car that wears out one piece at a time—first the fuel pump, then the bearings, then the generator, everything breaking down to lead to the final indignity, dying too long. For the geriatrician, the *terra incognita* means on-the-job training. There are no guidelines; each day is a new venture. Easy rules are hard to come by, and every facile piece of advice should be suspect, because death and dying are really a big deal. They are not to be avoided nor neglected, but should be faced rationally and competently as well as compassionately. A patient's death, for the physician, is too often viewed as a "defeat."

In 1987, in an effort to bring some pattern to what I was doing, I kept a running record of all my patients who died that year. There were 97 of them, one every 3 or 4 days, aged 60 to 106. This relatively high number was less a reflection of my skill as a physician than the type of patient under my care at the Palo Alto Clinic. Frankly, very few of my physician partners were comfortable with old patients. To check on their life courses, I reviewed their charts at 6 months, 1 month, and 1 week before they died and recorded four features: mobility, cognition, pain, and continence. I divided my 97 into three further categories depending on where they died: at home (13), in a nursing home (51), or in the hospital (33). I reported these observations in my paper "The Trajectory of Dying," published in the *Journal of the American Geriatrics Society* (1).

My Stanford colleague Jim Fries came up with the phrase "compression of morbidity," which expresses the hope that when the final swoon comes, it will happen abruptly, like the bursting of a bubble (2). My paper showed that some of my patients' deaths reflected that bubble-like scenario, while others had a lamentable dying-by-inches and slow-moments script. Modern medicine has the power to determine which trajectory prevails.

The major issue is that modern technology has given us newfound capacity to sustain life, which can result in an inhumane corruption of the dying process. Death and dying are different today. It is certainly true that none of the 151 billion people who ever existed has survived. No single soul has escaped alive. One death per birth is a standard ratio. Not dying is not an option.

My principal problem with the issue of death and dying stems less from the technical ugliness with which it is too often admixed as from the fact that most early deaths are preventable. This is an enormous cultural issue that has profound societal implications. The first secret to relieving death anxiety is to live to be 100, full of life. Do not die too soon. Very few of us have had the chance to blow out 100 candles to date, but more will, particularly once the principles of Next Medicine are learned and routinely embraced. To reiterate: Aging is a self-fulfilling prophecy.

Socrates declared that the unexamined life is not worth living (3). As we become increasingly capable of examining life, we must examine death as well. Ignorance breeds fear, so as we diminish ignorance, our fear will also decrease. As we learn how to live, we will learn better how to die. Since our science is newly capable of answering Schrodinger's key inquiry, "What is life?" we, using the same tools, can confidently answer the corollary question, "What is death?"

## Folk Wisdom About Dying and Death

From the beginning, humankind has sought a relationship with death, but its randomness, cruelty, and obscurity have made it incomprehensible. Twenty-five hundred years ago, Epicurus taught that death was natural. He rejected any metaphysical component, particularly the idea of divine retribution after death (4). He taught that death, after all is said and done, is merely a redistribution of our matter into another form. Religion bundled creation and extinction myths, common to all cultures and infinite in variety—Nirvana, jihad, heaven, hell, purgatory, happy hunting ground, devils, angels, paradise, Inferno. *The End of Faith,* a book by Sam Harris, goes so far as to state that death, and the desire to explain this most elusive mystery, is really the fundamental reason behind the development of all religions (5).

The proposition that we face a tormented afterlife is, I submit, a shameless attack on humanity's dignity and essence. It represents the tortured logic of original sin, which burdens humankind with a built-in guilt trip arbitrated by a self-serving church. We all suffer mightily under this awful miscarriage of truth, which is an insult to our nature and to the powerful ethics that speak to us from nature. The Golden Rule and Kant's Categorical Imperative (act in such a way that your action can be a universal law), neither of which involve any divine inspiration, spring from millions of years of humanity's striving for the collective right.

In times past, most deaths were those of young people. The pain of death varies inversely with age, and the death of any child is horrible. Now, however, 75% of deaths occur after 75 years of age. And certainly this percentage will increase further, and with that the terror caused by dying too soon. The human potential is a mandate, and staying its course is the worthiest of commitments. Norman Cousins advised us to "Worry less about life after death. Worry instead about assuring life before death" (6). I endorse this, fervently.

Still, our temporariness offends. As George Santayana said, "I know we all have to die someday, but I'm just hoping that there may be an exception made in my case" (7). But think of animals: they have no need for metaphysical exit theories; they live and then die. Our egos demand more, but our egos rarely coincide with reality. As we reconcile our egos with nature, peace and harmony will prevail. Mark Twain said it best: "I do not fear death. I had been dead for billions of years before I was born and had not suffered the slightest inconvenience from it" (8).

## Defining Dying and Death

Just as science has allowed us to define a healthy life, complete with metrics, we are getting close to being able to define a healthy death, with its own set of metrics. Employing our personal calendar of 100 years of life, our health span, we can presume that our birth certificate has an expiration date on it—I say 100 years after birth. But like a driver's license, the health license can be renewed. For some, the 100th birthday is not the final destination, the adieu. Hypothetically, however, the century mark is a handy date to increase focus on one's death.

I assume that on my 100th birthday or thereafter I will agree that my life's potential has been wrung out. When basic functions are lost, when flow ebbs, and when joy no longer illumines a Christmas morning or a sunset exalts, then life will have reached its terminus. The birthday party, the last supper, will be a major bash. When I awake on March 21, 2030, I will have had my last food and water, and I will die soon thereafter, on cue. When science writer Otto Segerberg surveyed a large number of centenarians, he found that they faced death with great equanimity (9): it had lost its sting.

Defining dying and death is a trickier business than it might seem, as we see from cases of legal wrangling over people in persistent vegetative states and irreversible comas. Interventions by increasingly sophisticated life-support systems mask the time-tested signs of death: absence of breath or heartbeat. Now, the cessation of function by the whole brain, the brain stem, or the seat of self-efficacy, the neocortex, are all part of the definition.

In the typical death one organ or system fails first—heart, lung, liver, pancreas, kidney—leading eventually to the terminal cascade, when all the homeo-dynamically conformed systems collapse in a rush, much like "The Wonderful One-Hoss Shay" in the poem by Oliver Wendell Holmes (10) that ends:

> You see, of course, if you're not a dunce,
> How it went to pieces all at once,
> —All at once, and nothing first,
> —Just as bubbles do when they burst.

## Tame Death, Wild Death

Dan Callahan, emeritus director of the Hastings Institute, is one of our most respected and effective commentators on death. His books *Setting Limits* (11) and, more recently, *The Troubled Dream of Life: In Search of a Peaceful Death* (12) are masterworks of caring introspection into life's end. Callahan helps clarify death by distinguishing "tame death" from "wild death," terms that he borrowed from the French historian Philippe Aries. "Tame death" was the norm for most of human history—it was in plain sight. For thousands of years, death was precipitated largely by infection on top of poor nutrition. Such deaths came suddenly, often in large numbers. Medicine was of no avail. People sought comfort in church doctrine, which in my view exploited death for its own purposes. The tame death has historically been a shared experience, usually a public display and ritual, a familiar simplicity, often combined with a reasoned anticipation of the distribution of worldly goods, almost a casual indifference. I recall Lewis Thomas's portrait of certain wild animals, which when being killed act as though they were only spectators at their own dying.

"Wild death" is modern—the means of death have often been surrendered to institutions and technology, externalized. Aries and Callahan describe the wild death as an ugly biological event, hidden and dirty, fear-filled, too often denied, out of sight, and uncomfortably sanitized. Dead bodies are not usually grieved over, but rather recalled in "memorial" ceremonies. Callahan lays most of the blame for the too-frequent scenario of "wild death" at the hands of the medical profession. Wild death is an exclusive byproduct of high-tech medicine. The tameness of low-tech dying has been eclipsed by ghastly scenarios like the pitiful Terry Schiavo case, which was what I would call death pornography. We lose a lot to machines. We are dehumanized by tubes and electricity. We lose our primal nature when surrogacy is inserted into death. As former Colorado governor Richard Lamm asked perceptively in his 2003 book, *The Brave New World of Health Care*: "Are we prolonging life or prolonging death?"(13)

The fact that Current Medicine expropriated death and dying for its own purposes, like the church in older times, is most grotesque. The variety of gadgets and tubes that we have developed ultimately serve to insulate the body from its own dying process. We can breathe, cause a heart to beat, cleanse the blood, arrest bleeding. Callahan laments medicine's general unfamiliarity with death and its lack of understanding of death's place in medical theory. The low-tech use of feeding tubes seems to represent the least offensive intrusion into life's ebb. However, a feeding tube is nonetheless a medical intervention and should be regarded as such. As with other tubes, a feeding tube prohibits the body from participating in its own natural conclusion.


## Extraordinary Measures: Utility and Futility

Because of my pro-aging orientation, I have taken issue with some of Callahan's counsel about not spending too much money on old people and their dying process. I insist that age is not the disqualifier—life quality is. Some people are so immersed in futile lives at younger ages that taking extraordinary measures is simply wrong for them. I have participated in numerous debates, insisting that functionality rather than age should be the guide when it comes to the use of life-extending technology.

I have previously recorded my experience with a lovely 88-year-old patient whose cardiac arrest resulted in a flail chest, a mechanically unstable and fatal condition, after resuscitation efforts. At my direction, and with the family's concurrence, we persisted, despite clear problems, in major supportive efforts in the ICU, and she eventually walked out of the hospital and lived a fully participatory year thereafter. When we consider when and whether to take extraordinary measures to continue life, we have to take into account the concept of medical futility, that situation in which the medical system, for all its wonders, is powerless to prevent the inevitable.

Defining futility seems as though it should be a slam-dunk, but the vagaries of recent biology make such categorization imprecise at best. Futility is a large and complex issue. When the prospect of a cure or of marked improvement is lacking, and there is no logical chance of restoring quality life, then futility should be recognized and deferred to. Several monographs exist to provide guidance in determining futility. The prime participant should be given sufficient data to yield a fair prognostic guide. In most cases, reasonable people looking at the data can reach a cessation-of-treatment decision.

But up to that point, more than data are needed. I have elsewhere recorded my experience with Mother Teresa in her convent in Calcutta on Palm Sunday morning in 1987. Within a half hour of arriving at Howrah railway station, my wife and I were seated with this almond-faced gentlewoman whose memory we all revere. I began, "I am an American physician devoutly concerned and daily consumed with the issues of how we decide how much to do and how much not to do for old and dying persons." Mother Teresa answered, "Dr. Bortz, don't worry about that, just love them." I could have responded to any other advice, but "Don't worry about that" is not in my repertoire. She suggested that I visit her Home for the Dying in the southern part of Calcutta, which I did the next morning. I spent most of the day in my green smock with the other volunteers. I was very self-conscious and ill at ease. I visited with the staff and absorbed their concerns. My clumsiness as a bedside nurse was humbling. I tried to feed porridge to several of the dying and managed to get more on me than in them. I recognized that the next day they would be gone. The great majority of the people at the home died, the men from tuberculosis, the women from sepsis, and they were given only token medical care. A nickel's worth of penicillin could have saved most. Mother Teresa's calculation was that if they were saved that day and discharged to the streets of Calcutta, they would be back again shortly. Meanwhile, there were 300,000 similar others waiting to enter. Seen in this light, it was clear that love was the appropriate therapy, a measure both ordinary and extraordinary.

We should always take the extraordinary measure of being honest with the dying person and his or her loved ones, to comfort always. Callahan recalls Tolstoy's powerful story of the death of Ivan Ilyich, a middle-aged bureaucrat dying of what I might guess was stomach cancer (14). Tolstoy wrote: "The worst torment was the lie, this lie that for some reason was accepted by everyone, that he was only sick and not dying, and that if he would only remain calm and take care of himself everything would be fine. He suffered because they lied to him, forced him to take part in this deception, which degraded the formidable and solemn act of his own death."

I recall vividly, in my training years, the deception that was foisted upon patients with a fatal prognosis. Shameful and usually all-too-transparent charades were perpetrated in the name of "saving Mom from the bad news." Fortunately this grim game is no longer sanctioned.

We often talk about the high cost of dying. Estimates of how high it is vary, but no matter how low an estimate we accept, it is too high. Dying should be cheap. My formula for a good death is no tubes, no pain, and no loneliness, all inexpensive features. It is only when the medical system intrudes into the scene that costs soar.

Consider this story of a well-intentioned neighbor who was chicken-sitting our daughter Danna's flock and found one to be badly tattered. Reflexively, she called the vet, who ordered a CAT scan without thinking. When Danna heard of this she blew her top. She considered the $1,600 bill an absurd excess, particularly if you follow the logic and ask what you are going to do with the information once you have it. Now we are trying to teach our medical students, house staff, and attending staff to be more sensitive to the costs associated with many of the orders we write for hospital patients as they die. Consider whether the technological imperative is worth the cost, whether it is reasonable, rather than reacting reflexively.

## Taming Wild Death

It is essential that the individual maintain control of medicine's role at the end of life. The wild death scenario is too real, but it is avoidable, provided the individual has thought through the particulars and practicalities in advance. The issue of advance directives, or living wills, is mandatory in any rational approach to death and dying. The most important person in the event must have primary say in how it plays out. Unfortunately, only a small percentage of people have executed one.

But as fundamental as the directive is, it is insufficient. There is just too much mischief involved in dying. I have been witness to thousands of deaths, many with prior directives in place, only to see the stated intention overridden either by ignorance or by neglect. This means that thorough backup instructions must be available; the family and the medical caregiver must be intimately involved and committed to honoring the advance directive.

When the climactic moment arrives, the question of "how" is of paramount concern. A system-wide, not a piece-by-piece, death is to be desired. One hopes for an abrupt last breath. Choosing to stop taking nourishment is the logical option when declaring one's intention to die. Suicide and euthanasia are other options, but both have problems and issues associated with them. The abruptness of suicide is a stark jolt to loved ones and friends. Euthanasia, which I philosophically favor, still lacks adequate legal safeguards. The cessation of eating and drinking makes sense. One cannot choose to stop breathing, which is hypothetically appealing, or to stop one's heart from beating.

So, stopping eating and drinking is the prime strategy. Georgetown bioethicist Joanne Lynn is our leading theorist in this area (15). She has published extensively on the appropriateness and naturalness of this election. She assures us that the resulting death is gentle and distress-free. Someone must pay attention to keeping the mouth moist, but even this requirement is very benign. Withdrawal of food and fluid results in death in several days to several weeks. There is no drama, only increasing stupor and lethargy as the body slowly turns itself off. Gradually, waste materials accumulate in the blood and the mineral balances are disordered, leading to system failure.

Taking control of the dying process includes deciding where to die. The hospice movement has been a huge help in encouraging people to die at home. Home is where self-efficacy lives. The hospital is a hostile zone for maintaining self-efficacy.

It is the institutional setting for most wild deaths. I would question how many of us, in a dispassionate objective moment, would choose to die in a hospital. True, many people, out of a sense of consideration for the inconvenience and emotional burden placed upon family, might seek to die in the detached way. But when we are able to define death objectively and anticipate it, it appears much less formidable.

As I approach a dying patient, one of my most insistent assurances is that the person will be kept fully franchised until the last flutter. As Bandura would say, the answer to the question, "When shall I give up my self-efficacy?" is an emphatic "Never!"

Pain, of course, is a dominant player in our fear of death and dying. Fear of pain can grow into an obsession, but our technical competence is now such that the dying person can be absolutely assured that pain should not be his or her burden. The dying person should have absolute control over pain management. My father adopted a Browning exhortation, "Then welcome each rebuff that turns earth's smoothness rough, that bids each man not sit, nor stand, but go" (16). Rage at the dying of the light, but when the embers are clearly dimmed, then accept the grace that accompanies the well-lived life.

Having sorted through my myriad experiences with dying persons, I have codified my personal strategy—very simply: no pain, no tubes, and no loneliness. The first two of these responsibilities I welcome. The third strategy is one that all of us need to grapple with.

## Sending Out Ripples

I love the comment that the size of your funeral depends upon the weather. Irving Yalom, distinguished Stanford psychiatrist and an authority on death anxiety, recently wrote *Staring at the Sun*, in which he offers an alluring image of ripples representing the eventual emanation of life's work (17). "Ripples" acknowledges the temporal nature of the physical body, but asserts the continuation of life's energies. Death, in this interpretation, is more than merely the shedding of our corporeal ballast; it is the persistence of our energy field. The ripples concept effectively answers the primal fear of oblivion, the thought that when I die, everything about me is gone. Not so: ripples remain and endure. This is the same idea as the butterfly effect, Francis Thompson's "thou canst not stir a flower without troubling of a star" (18), the First Law of Thermodynamics— the conservation of energy. Rippling exalts Mozart, Buddha, Aristotle, Christ, Einstein, and Darwin, whose life energies persist and penetrate today more profoundly than they did when they were alive. Similarly, even the most modest among us leaves ripples behind.

We can imagine the body as a multifaceted antenna that over the course of a lifetime catches a century's worth of energy packets, repackages them, and redistributes them as our legacy. We are a prism made of CHNOPS refracting our life's rays in different patterns. As my CHNOPS returns to its original random distribution, my energies reside in Yalom's congenial concept of ripples, which I hope will send out their effects in a genial, benevolent way.

I propose that the concept of Grace, however it is defined, should be the anticipated end state of a life nobly lived, the full realization of our individual potential. It is our best reach to the denial of oblivion (19).

# Framing Next Medicine | 12

The replacement paradigm of Next Medicine requires a rigorous functional definition, ratified by the new science of health. Just as the colonists took a while to frame the Constitution to undergird their statement of autonomy, Next Medicine must build an administrative framework to put its precepts into operation.

It is critical that the structure match the function—the nurture and nature must reinforce one another. The administrative structures of Current Medicine are manifestly perverse and are in essence the very origin of the elaborate dysfunctional symptoms I have described. I assert that as the new structure and function of Next Medicine are implemented they will eradicate the cost, injustice, danger, corruption, inefficiency, and irrelevancy of Current Medicine.

For a reference point I return to medicine's mission of affirming and assuring human potential. Medical science has identified our potential as 100 healthy years. Robert Butler, first Director of the National Institute on Aging, commented: "We haven't found any biologic reason not to live to 100" (1). Most of the new paradigm's work consists in ensuring that we reach this noble goal. Current Medicine's elaborate list of symptoms is proof that it is inadequate and needs to be replaced. The glitch in the steady lengthening of longevity is a sad testament to its failings. The gross mismatch between our biology, our nature,

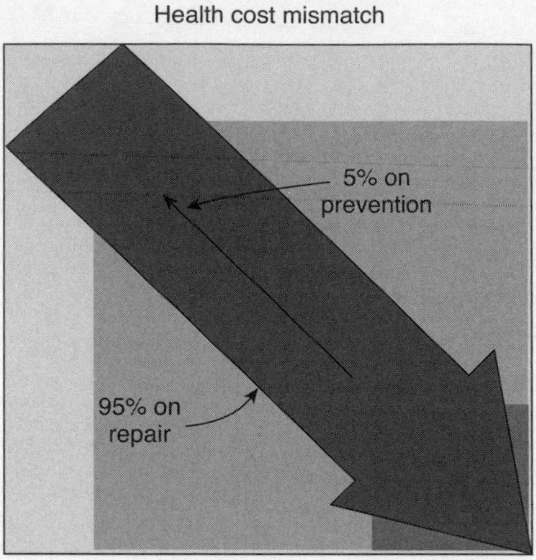

Health cost mismatch

**Figure 12.1**  Mismatch (95% repair/5% prevention).

and our current nurture, capitalism, is the diagnosis. For remedy, we need a
new administrative scaffolding to support the new paradigm of health.

The newly available equation of the determinants of health is a powerful tool
for designing the new infrastructure. As we solve the equation to seek 100 healthy
years, we identify four exponentials. Two are changeable (choice), and two are
immutable (fate). Fortunately, the two more quantitatively significant determinants—accidents and maintenance—yield to intervention. As we've seen,
Medicine's intervention capacity is divided into repair and prevention, with repair
representing 95% and more of our investment in health care. (Figure 12.1)

Let's recall Nobel laureate Sydney Brenner's observation at a Stanford
symposium in 2004: "You can't know everything. But you don't have to know
everything. Only enough" (2). Enough for what? Enough to put the health
equation into operation. We do not need to know every speck of our structure
and function. The Human Genome Project, for instance, has amassed a trainful
of information, but very little knowledge that would help us solve our equation.
All the information we need for 100 healthy years is this: first, to be sure that the
interaction between the organism, us, and our environment is ideally tuned
and modulated—not too much, not too little (the Golden Mean again)—so that
our adaptive phenotypic plasticity is optimal. Second, we must be assured of
sufficient supply of our two fuels, food and oxygen. Again, not too much, but
enough. Our historical food shortages have been replaced by excess, by worldwide obesity (globesity). Oxygen sufficiency is not limited by environmental
availability but by a default in our organism's transport system. Assuring our
potential depends on our acting on this minimal "enough" knowledge.

## Politics

A 2010 Kaiser Family Foundation survey indicated that 61% of the American public favors structural reform of health care now (3). The status quo is not an option, and as of this writing the United States teeters on the edge of health care reform. Ezekiel Emanuel says that change happens when there is general acknowledgment of a big problem, shared agreement about needs, a champion, and finally a transformative political event, all of which are now in evidence (4).

Perhaps the biggest endorsement of the urgent need for change comes from the fiscal side. Peter Orszag, now the head of the Federal Office of Management and Budget, commented at a Stanford health care symposium in March 2009 that unless we get a handle on our current health care mess fast, we can forget the rest of the country's business (5). President Obama and top congressional leaders of both parties share this sense of urgency. Perhaps never before in American history has there been such a confluence of previously competing interests. Shared values and shared fears and shared knowledge engender new agreement. Organizations as diverse as the AMA, AARP, the Chamber of Commerce, unions, and industry are all addressing the current crisis.

In addressing the challenge we cannot be timid. Incrementalism cannot work. Winston Churchill said that chasms cannot be crossed by progressive leaps. To establish the new structural paradigm of Next Medicine, we must return to First Principles. Unlike the failed Clinton proposal—all 1,342 pages of numbing words—the new paradigm's planks are simple, its blueprint self-evident: health instead of disease, prevention instead of repair, the individual as locus of control instead of the profession, and a structure that supports the new function.

## The Economists Comment

In 1963, invited by the Ford Foundation to extend his Nobel Prize-winning observations, economist Kenneth Arrow published his seminal paper "Uncertainty and the Welfare Economics of Medical Care" in the *American Economics Review* (6). This widely cited essay is credited as the origin of health economics. Its relevance seems to increase as time passes. A 2004 review of the article in the *Bulletin of the WHO* remarks how dramatically the medical marketplace has changed since the original publication, when the medical system was modest in all aspects, unlike today (7). Yet Arrow's underlying lesson concerns the efficient allocation of resources between the market and non-market constituencies. The complexity and speed of changes occurring in medical science challenge the contention that the medical market is self-regulating. The resultant out-of-control cost overruns seem to nullify this utopian claim.

However, Clayton Christensen of the Harvard Business School claims that an economic model is "industry agnostic," and that the medical system is not unique, as many claim (8). But to make his case, he recommends great disruption, a revolution. Central to his argument is that a business model can work if the product is changed from repair to prevention, so that the primary customer is not the sickest person among us, but the great majority with minor issues. He in effect changes the vector of the ecology of medical care from the right margin of the diagram in Figure 4.1 (intensive care) to the left (home and community). Intel founder Andy Groves' "left shift" proposal—from the medical center to the home—is similar (9). Christensen argues for more and cheaper care and more convenient care. He advocates a return to lower-level care systems. He is critical of regulatory restrictions that impede downward delegation of authority; he is an enthusiast of medical kiosks and paramedical personnel. He feels that in general there is substantial overshooting of personal competency, with too many invasive cardiologists and not enough health educators—maybe in the neighborhood of 20 educators per interventionist for evidence of return on investment. He recommends a realignment of many of the societal and political forces that constrain experimentation. He feels that the FDA and NIH are largely protective of the status quo and do not encourage experimentation. Like others, he feels that Kaiser, Mayo, and VA hospital models that provide trans-system integrated care are the gold standard. Prevention must be embraced as a primary strategy, and self-management as a key strategy. I welcome this perspective, since it endorses Peter Orszag's prediction that the breakthroughs in health care will come not from gleaming laboratories but from the ledger sheets of economists. In his October 2008 lecture at Harvard Medical School, Orszag lobbied for greater attention to behavioral research in the creation of medical science policy (10).

Each year, one of my favorite days is a late June opportunity to lecture to the Summer Executive Program at the vaunted Stanford Business School. More than 130 CEOs, COOs, and HR executives congregate from all over the world—Dubai, Zürich, Tokyo, New York—for an intensive 5-week program (at a cost of $50,000 per student). They are there to get richer by absorbing pearls of wisdom from the famous faculty members.

Mine is the very first lecture. "What is the most important asset in your life? Who owns that asset?" These basic questions frame the discussion as I hope to persuade these captains of capitalism that health is far and away the most important capital asset. But to bank this asset requires self-service; it cannot be delegated to a clerk or accountant. The term "healthwealth" seems right. I proceed to go through my determinants of health material for my capitalist students, as recounted in Chapter 7.

As the new paradigm of Next Medicine is implanted, it is critical that the economic incentive plan be sturdy. We are fortunate that we need no extra funds for the reformulation; in fact, we should have money left over. The surplus, which I cheerfully estimate at $1 trillion per year, would then be available for a national educational priority, which most claim to be among our greatest needs.

In the March 26, 2009, issue of the *New York Review of Books*, Harvard Nobel-winning economist Amartya Sen asks whether a New Capitalism is appropriate, our present model being possibly "exhausted" (11). His topic was also that of an international conference held in Paris in January 2009. The central issue is whether our current model of capitalism is such a byproduct of the "breathless pursuit of profit" that it encourages social imbalance. The challenge of former labor secretary Robert Reich's "super capitalism," like Sen's, has much to do with the medical care system's compact with society (12). Echoing Arrow's sentiment that health care has a larger agenda than quick profit, they ask whether the social mission is also the economic one. All of this surrounds the question of whether a healthy democracy, rather than fearing regulatory oversight, actually depends on it. If a democracy is burdened by stockholder equity, it becomes overrun with neglect and misbehavior, as seen in the present business sector meltdown. A similar scenario beckons for the medical system.

Sen recognizes the experience of China, which until 1979 had universal coverage for its citizens. After becoming infected with the capitalist lust, it revoked that coverage, leading to a shortening of life expectancy and increased infant mortality. On the other hand, Kerala, the Indian state to its south, has retained its universal coverage and despite a markedly lower economic profile, it outperforms China.

## Physician Charter

In a 2001 *JAMA* article, Hal Sox, former editor of the *Annals of Internal Medicine*, set out the three fundamental principles of the Physician Charter for the new millennium: "The first of the three principles is the primacy of patient welfare. The second is patient autonomy. In this view the center of patient care is not in the physician's office or a hospital. It is where people live their lives, in the home and in the workplace. There, patients make their daily choices that determine their health." The last of the three principles is that of social justice: the profession is called upon to promote a fair distribution of healthcare resources (13,14). In essence, these precepts constitute the basis of Next Medicine's contract with society.

The issue of professional oversight of patient responsibility has come into brighter focus with a plan in West Virginia, wherein the benefits of Medicaid recipients who fail to adhere to medical advisories are reduced or eliminated. This raises the fundamental issue of fairness for patients who seemingly are discriminated against by "conditions that are beyond their control" (15). But what about the patient who smokes after heart surgery or drinks after a liver transplant? These issues raise the concern that we are giving an actuarial value to behavior. This places the physician's professionalism in conflict with traditional values. Is it infringement on a patient's autonomy? It is notable that WHO does not hire smokers. Is this fair? A survey discussed in a July 2006 *Wall Street Journal* article reveals that 53% of Americans feel that it is fair for insurers to charge more for people who maintain an unhealthy lifestyle (15 A).

We all applauded Massachusetts' wonderfully created insurance plan covering all its citizens (16). The consequent $2 billion deficit, however, burdened the state budget to the extent that welfare recipients may no longer receive subsidies for their heating bills.

In a lecture at Harvard Law School in June 2008, Alain Enthoven quoted Charles Sills's lecture of 30 years before: "The most important social convention mankind has invented is the creation of incentives so that public goods become private interests. Incentives must align. Imposing a solution without remedying the incentives regularly fails" (17).

The topic of the civics of health is unlikely to draw much of a crowd to a lecture, even among those with a medical interest. But it is through civics that health is put into practice. Civics is the area of human endeavor concerned with the allocation of common resources, with empowerment and the gratification of needs. It is the area where individual rights and community obligations intersect.

The civics of health has a long history. The Greek ethos rested on three fundamental principles. The first was that we are all equal, morally and physically, in having an array of shared basic survival needs. These needs create a moral imperative for a good society. Two, we vary in significant ways in our talents and merits, and these differences present a claim on distribution. Variance in merits and effort represents a just principle for individual claims. Three, since we all benefit from being members of the community, we have a duty to contribute a proportionate share to that community. The polis would have had problems with our present structure in that it lacks *civitas*, the acknowledgment of egalitarianism, of a sense of sharing, expressed in representative community councils, which insist that the citizen must have a moral compass.

Social justice emerged as the resolution of the three principles. Aristotle developed a code of balance in negotiating these claims (18). The first two, common needs and different talents, are generally acknowledged, yet it is in the third proposition, the responsibility of all to share with those who received less in "the lottery of nature," that uncertainty arises. Aristotle also mentioned that the good condition of the people is a more significant principle than the good condition of property. As Dostoevsky proclaimed in *The Brothers Karamazov*, "We are all responsible for one another" (19).

The process Plato described in *The Republic*, of transforming asceticism to hedonism, of going from "a healthy city to a flawed city," evolved rapidly (20). Asceticism was an emphasis on non-material values, a renunciation of physical pleasures, simplicity, self-denial, and arduous, purposeful discipline. Hedonism is asceticism's alter-ego. When asceticism and a material form of hedonism, acquisitiveness, collided centuries ago, the world began to change, and our culture is a product of that change.

## Capitalism and Next Medicine

We live at a moment of collision between our nature and capitalism, and our Kuhnian reformulation must prominently acknowledge this collision. Our goal must be to put these two bodies in orbit around each other so that they do not keep crashing. In his book *The Cultural Contradictions of Capitalism*, social scientist Daniel Bell claims that the seeds of capitalism were planted in 16th-century Europe (21). At that moment, the two forces of asceticism and acquisitiveness became yoked to generate capitalism. This bespoke the exploration of the "endless frontier," leading to the fundamental transformation of nature, with humankind becoming an agent of accelerated change.

The ascetic dimension of early capitalism was quickly submerged in the demands of acquisitiveness. Thomas Aquinas, the Dominican priest of the 13th century, wrote that "the desire for money knows no limits" (22). Capitalism is the economic strategy that much of global society has chosen as its economic engine. It has withstood challenges from dictatorships and from communism. Bell further outlines the extraordinary dynamism and boundless energy of capitalism. Capitalism offers the prospect that a rising tide of an affluent society will lift all boats. The gross disparities in health care suggest that this does not always happen: the tides are too unpredictable, flooding some and stranding others.

The market has assumed the primary role in arbitrating societal functions. For many, enough is never enough; "more" is the commandment. When John D.

Rockefeller was asked once how much more money he desired, he replied, "One more dollar" (23). Technology and the credit card economy seem to encourage a culture of instant gratification, a dulling of responsibility, and a diminishing sense of equity.

So Bell insists, as did the Greeks, on the differentiation between needs, which are biological and legitimate, and wants, which are psychological and without the same degree of legitimacy. He points to John Rawls, author of *A Theory of Justice*, the primary text on political philosophy, as the outstanding recent advocate for a theory of distributive justice and a rationalization of democracy's competing claims (24). The distribution rule is that some persons are better off, but no one should be worse off; that is, those with more should strive toward a general equity.

In the polis, the private and public interest are in constant struggle. Bell cites Isaiah Berlin, who reconciles personal freedoms and individual liberties with a community function: "Sometimes it is necessary to forgo some personal freedom to obtain the freedom of others" (25). Therefore, Bell recommends "the public household" as an alternative to the domestic household and a market economy that can, in his view, mediate the intersection between private need and public good. Bell notes that our natural needs are best satisfied in a small community, whereas a larger arena with no rules has difficulty resolving competing claims. The public good is more strongly recognized in a small community. Increasing size invariably isolates people and erodes sensitivity. We must therefore redraw the boundaries of the "community" as we begin to make Next Medicine policy.

## Commonhealth

In 1968, Garrett Hardin published a famous essay, "The Tragedy of the Commons," in *Science* (26). He took his image from one proposed in 1852 by William Forster Lloyd, an Oxford political economist, who wondered why the cattle in the publicly owned pastures of England were so puny and stunted compared with those raised in the adjacent private fields. Lloyd posited that the use of the common pastures, full of self-interest, cheating, and competition, had become corrupted. When individualism invades the commons, degradation follows. Hardin extended his theme to include James Madison's 1788 quote: "If men were angels, no government would be necessary" (27). In a world in which resources are limited, a single non-angel in the commons spoils the environment for all. "Ruin is the destruction toward which all men rush, each pursuing his own best interest in a society that believes in the freedom of the commons," Hardin writes. In this connection, Hardin notes Hegel's statement that "freedom is the recognition of necessity" (28). Hardin's fundamental argument is that any culture in its early development provides maximum potential for everyone's growth, but as time passes, the commons becomes crowded, and competition and cheating intervene and erode the early freedoms. This powerful metaphor, similar to that of a crowded lifeboat, justifies the government's role in overseeing and managing the commons. Abraham Lincoln said, "Why should we have government?" He answered his own question: "The legitimate object of government is to do for the people whatever they need to have done but which they cannot do, at all, or cannot do so well, for themselves in their separate and individual capacities" (29).

In his 1975 article in the *New England Journal of Medicine*, "Protecting the Commons: Who Is Responsible?" (30) Howard Hiatt also uses the metaphor of the town pasture. Hiatt, who was the dean of the School of Public Health at Harvard, argued that medical care is the contemporary equivalent of the commons on which increasing competitive demands are being made, and he identified certain characteristics of medicine that contribute to the drain. First is the age-old principle of medical practice, "Do everything possible for the individual patient." Second is the fact that much of what is done is of little value.

Health, Hiatt argued, is not the exclusive province of medicine. He made prominent mention of the excessive demands on the commons made by conditions that are potentially preventable, including many cancers. He pointed to nutrition, education, and housing as corollary, but seldom identified, determinants of health, and he advocated physicians' ongoing participation in a larger dialogue, emphasizing the role of rigorous, flexible pilot experiments seeking a more rational allocation of resources.

In a 2007 *JAMA* article, "Managing Medical Resources: Return to the Commons?" Chris Cassel and T. E. Brennan of the American Board of Internal Medicine expressed concern that physicians traditionally focus on the scientific particulars of their profession and have little interest in administrative efficiency and cost issues (31). There is a disconnect between responsibility to the patient and to the health of the commons. They particularly identify the lack of a forum, a representative body, where various constituencies may congregate in a virtual commons, where the physician and the patient and the administrative apparatus can debate, discuss, and allocate resources. Several major medical organizations have coalesced around the proposal for a Medical Charter in which, like the Hippocratic Oath, physicians may find common cause.

Mark Siegler of the University of Chicago has argued that the physician and the patient no longer play primary roles in the commons (32). The bankers now hold all the keys. The rules of a simple bioethical system have been overrun by the capitalistic demands of the landholder. The commons is no longer common. Democracy, government of, by, and for the people, has been degraded by common greed. Is medicine a sturdy partner in the American experiment in shared government, or has it been consumed by the rapaciousness of capitalistic enterprise? Has medicine lost its nobility of purpose and conduct?

Political discourse in America has focused almost exclusively on the question of who will pick up the tab for our health care costs. This narrow focus leaves us exposed on all the issues that lead up to the financial and administrative ones. We must commit to the ideal of Commonhealth. The individual, the medical profession, and society as a whole must adopt the new paradigm of Next Medicine.

## Implementing Commonhealth in Next Medicine

America has uniquely resisted government intrusion into its citizens' lives and has steadfastly accepted fragmentation and inefficiency as an acceptable tradeoff against further regulation. We have lacked social solidarity when it comes to matters of health, but we must accept an expanded government role in the restructure of health care delivery. We acknowledge the need for government involvement in national defense, education, and many regulatory actions. The lack of adequate oversight in the financial world is the basic reason for our current depression. The employer-based, private insurance model must go. In its place, we need a single-payer, para-governmental administrative structure that affirms the Commonhealth and aligns the incentives in its pursuit. Creating the administrative structure for the Commonhealth requires the muscle and reach of the federal government.

The new government entity must be insulated from political influences and must be assured of continued adequate funding. In my view, Medicare expansion should be used as the vehicle for providing universal coverage, but it must be an expansion with other features, such as mandatory not-for-profit status, which in effect erases the fee-for-service that defines Current Medicine and its repair fixation. Our new system of funding would immediately derail the private health insurers. They will be little mourned when replaced by an efficient, cheaper, integrated new system.

The future administrative apparatus will evolve rapidly but should include strict oversight and massively expanded and available outcome results. A group at the Rand Corporation has maintained an ongoing technology designed to measure not so much clinical results as personal satisfaction and choice (33). The National Health Board (not unlike the Federal Reserve Board model), as

White House chief of staff Rahm Emanuel has termed it, will oversee 12 regional health boards that will allocate dedicated tax dollars according to regularly adjusted criteria, reflecting the needs and practices of each region. These boards will represent professional and public interests.

Every citizen would have a choice of integrated delivery systems managed under the regional health boards. Participation by all would be mandated. The regional health boards will set standard operational guidelines. They will incentivize the development of multiple nonprofit HMOs such as Kaiser and Puget Sound, which are individually managed and compete with one another, like the Dutch system of managed competition. These health systems will be required to enroll all applicants and will operate within a global common budget with set, but adjustable, caps.

## HMO Revised

My suggestion that people should be rewarded for their health is a residue of a contract that my wife and I signed with our four children when we were young marrieds. In an effort to encourage school attendance, we promised our kids $50 each year if they never missed a day of school. I do not believe they ever missed a single one. Even if they had a fever, we reasoned that even if they were possibly contagious, this was actually a benefit to their schoolmates because it would stimulate their immune responsiveness. Beyond that, the bargain ingrained in them the notion of persistence despite minor symptoms. Life rewards what is done, not what is not done.

Certainly one of the most important current experiments in health care is the Kaiser medical system, established by Sidney Garfield in 1935 (34). The Kaiser Permanente Health plan has been the poster child for HMOs since its inception. Their pervasive radio and TV ads preaching "Thrive" display their devotion to healthy living. I support this enthusiastically, yet I am disquieted by their seeming inability to capitalize on their prevention strategy. I challenged their CEO, George Halvorson, on this. "Wait a little longer," he told me. What he meant was that their electronic medical record system, now near completion, has lacked the ability to display return on investment until now. With greatly expanded information technology and integrated systems, they will soon be able to affirm major cost/benefit advantage (23). Capitalism should work *for* health rather than against it.

An informal progress report from Kaiser's Hawaii complex, issued on November 20, 2008, concerned a pilot study that they had developed for patients with the "terrible triad" of congestive heart failure, coronary artery disease, and diabetes. These three separately are terrible, but together they are extremely ominous. The Hawaii Kaiser team created the trial program using their electronic record-keeping system, which informed the patient and the medical team of any possible change in status. Early warning was their goal. Within 6 months of initiation of the protocol, hospitalization rates fell more than 65% and emergency room visits by 34%.

A similar team approach by Kaiser in Southern California, called "Healthy Bone," reduced hip fracture rates in 620,000 people by 37% to 50% by means of a systematic focus on prevention. On the open market, a hip fracture costs $80,000, so the cost savings are immense. I eagerly await extension of these experimental programs to the Kaiser system at large. The cost savings should translate promptly to cheaper premiums and thereby a competitive marketing advantage. I expect the maturing of the Kaiser example and its quick extension to the rest of the health care system.

I have a deep interest in Kaiser's success, because in my view they embody most of the Next Medicine paradigm. But their proof of concept awaits further development of their electronic medical records, which will provide the necessary cost/benefit data that will dominate Next Medicine. The manifest advantages of an HMO system will emerge.

Are lifestyles susceptible to actuarial analysis? Behavioral anomalies cost lots of money and are changeable, so why not? A new, integrated health care system would be the ideal vehicle for introducing a vast preventive strategy. Primary care physicians and their physician-extender colleagues will constitute the backbone of the medical service providers. The roles of the specialists and subspecialists will recede as primary care and prevention are augmented and rewarded. All physicians will be salaried by their governing board, with incentive bonuses for documented superior outcomes. Fee-for-service will become a distant memory. Beyond the guaranteed standard benefits of office and home visits, hospitalization, and other ancillary services, individuals will be free to purchase additional services and amenities. The cost of these concierge services will not be tax-deductible.

The immense savings generated by such a simplified administrative proposal is in the range of hundreds of billions of dollars. Whether the new system employs a dedicated value-added tax (VAT) or simply expands the Medicare tax system would be decided in Washington. The point is that we are already spending such a huge slice of the GDP on health care that this proposed restructuring should provide great amounts of capital for other social purposes. Increased health literacy will inform and encourage the individual's involvement in his or her personal health trajectory. The expert patient, personal efficacy, and individual responsibility will prevail.

Implementing Next Medicine requires three major building materials: information, opportunity, and incentives: I-O-I. Information is essential for the paradigm shift. The replacement model must have proven numbers, experimental confirmation, and expert testimonials. Faith in platitudes is an insufficient basis for the kind of upheaval that is called for. Emphasis should be placed on expanding electronic records. The home computer and health monitors will be the centerpieces of self-care and improved self-efficacy.

Second, we must have the opportunity to exploit our health competence. For this we need time and space. In this frenzied world, we need to build in sufficient time to be healthy. And we need the space, the parks, the trails, the open lands, that contribute to health. Third, we need to build incentives for health (and disincentives for sickness). Similar to Theodosius Dobzhansky's insistence that nothing in biology makes sense except in the light of evolution (35), nothing in Medicine, Disease Medicine, Health Medicine, or Next Medicine makes sense except in the light of capitalism. It defines our culture.

## Information, Opportunity, Incentive: I-O-I

Most agree that health illiteracy is one of the most important aspects, if not the most important aspect, of our health challenge. Health illiteracy belongs at the top of the list of principal causes of death. Most sickness, including AIDS, heart disease, and many forms of cancer, is preventable. The best vaccine against ignorance is information.

Since health is our most important asset, it should surely occupy a prominent slot in school programs, beginning in kindergarten. The fact that there are probably a hundred times more physicians (sickness doctors) than health educators is backwards.

Our science base is much farther along in understanding the hard sciences of physics and chemistry than it is in the soft science of behavioral medicine. Recall Arthur Kornberg's remark to me at that Stanford lecture, "Because, Dr. Bortz, there is no science in behavior." This is no longer tolerable. True, we can know nature, but we cannot change it. But we can know nurture, and, critically, we *can* change it. Fortunately, nurture is the more quantitatively important determinant of health.

Our society has massively over-committed financial resources to a misshapen Current Medicine and massively under-committed to education. We have the opportunity to redress this by redirecting funds, mega-billions, to education at all levels. Our society would reap immense rewards, and not coincidentally reach for our potential by pursuing the Commonhealth.

In our paradigm shift, we will newly recognize the health educator. This is different from the MD, someone organic to the community, narrowly trained for a more targeted role, and cheaper, much cheaper, but most important, probably more effective. I feel strongly that the health adviser's ability to influence good adherence to a healthy lifestyle is more substantial than that of the high-profile physician.

Several years ago, in Vietnam, I had the opportunity to witness the high theater of Professor Alain Carpentier, a heart surgeon from Paris, who would fly into the country with his staff and, in a space of a few days, operate on a dozen or more children with deformed heart valves as a result of earlier rheumatic fever. His results are outstanding. Meanwhile, upstairs in the same hospitals in Hanoi and Saigon, the wards were filled with children with acute rheumatic fever, the result of an inefficient primary care system, which could eliminate the strep throat origin of rheumatic fever with a few pennies' worth of penicillin. Carpentier gets the headlines, but the health educator preaching prophylaxis is also a hero. Such examples multiply by the millions worldwide. While the experts exalt the miracles of the medical-industrial complex, preventive strategies belong in homes and neighborhoods. We need a vast supply of health promoters. The benefits they will bring will surely more than justify the expense.

## The Greening of Next Medicine

In the transition to Next Medicine, government should create policies that promote health. We need a political philosophy that pervades all segments of government, legislation, and fiscal policy. The government deserves much credit for its role in tobacco control. Its involvement, while far from ideal, was essential in the reallocation of agricultural subsidies. Such an aggressive advocacy role is easily converted into policy. There is now a common zeal for environmental protection, which is supplementary to health and the human potential. Increased federal involvement in ensuring healthy food is a logical pursuit. A George Will column in the *Washington Post* on March 6, 2009, linked our marginal health status with a politically driven subsidy for corn and the consequent glut of bad nurture (36), which writer Michael Pollan calls "overfed and undernourished" (37). One in five American meals is eaten in cars, resulting in the anomaly that gas stations make more money from food and cigarettes than from gas. This is grossly inconsistent with the Commonhealth and possibly has as much to do with the nation's health as all the country's cardiologists.

The connection between a healthy environment and a healthy people is a central facet of Hellenic political philosophy. Our legislators would do well to re-read Plato and Aristotle. The Greeks embraced the truth and beauty of nature, and proclaimed that the body and its environment should exist in simple harmony. We can only be as healthy as our world, which is our home. Our home in turn becomes healthier as we ourselves are healthy. Not at all coincidentally, what happens to be good for our physical and mental well-being creates a healthy environment as well. Being a representative democracy means that all citizens are involved in the creation and maintenance of our Commonhealth.

On a societal level, we have seen gas crises precipitate wars, and global warming spur air-conditioner sales. Green forests disappear into plastic bags and deserts. The Nature Conservancy was a response to this loss. Health Conservancy is an allied cause. Green Health makes sense, since it combines the virtue of nature in both the environment and in health.

The Industrial Revolution precipitated a sharp decline in health and increased mortality. Clean air, pure water, and good nutrition were replaced by pollution, sugared beverages, and junk food. Our financial institutions sought quick gain and created instruments that are easily corruptible. The resulting price paid for all is harm to the Commonhealth. What if the medical system were used to build and create and grow instead of patching the broken pieces?

## Incentives and Disincentives

The shift to the Next Medicine paradigm must include intimate consideration of the financial implications. Even a casual dissection of the costs represented in hospital discharge data indicates that the spike on the right side of Figure 2.1, Distribution of Costs, is very amenable to preventive strategies. The largest single charge is from congestive heart failure, in the range of $50 billion per year. Add to this other cardiovascular conditions, such as myocardial infarction, and the total is $150 billion per year. Other notable disease categories are arthritis at $24 billion, back pain $18 billion, drug overdose $4 billion, AIDS $3.2 billion, and complications resulting from medical treatment $50 billion. I estimate that the combined clinical components of the disuse syndrome account for over 30% of the hospital charges.

But incentive does not mean pouring more capital into the current paradigm of Disease Medicine. Disease should not pay. Instead, we need to reformulate the value of health in the terms of capitalism, so that health pays.

Prevention before treatment is indisputably cost-effective. On the surface of it, it makes much more sense and seems more self-evident, but the reality is that disease pays big time, and millions of jobs are consecrated to disease. It has been estimated, for instance, that more people are employed by cancer than are killed by it.

The Medicare/Medicaid office is currently trying to deny hospitals reimbursement for readmissions for certain conditions, congestive heart failure chief among them. The logic is that if a good enough effort were expended the first time, there would be no need for re-confinement. Following this line of argument, what about curtailing payment for all preventable conditions? It is absurd to label a hospital's status based on its occupancy figures. Hospitals should be paid for their empty beds rather than for their full ones.

"Health equals fitness equals function equals productivity equals profit" seems to make more sense than "disease equals frailty equals dysfunction equals profit." Testimonials to the economic benefits of good health are everywhere. Corporate health expenses appear on stockholder reports, Starbucks pays more for health care than for coffee (38), and so on.

The average American spends $8,200 per year on health expenses. My friend Nico Pronk, prime biostatistician at Health Partners in Minneapolis, published a paper in *JAMA*, "Relation Between Modifiable Health Risks and Short-term Health Care Charges," in 1999, in which he surveyed 5,689 adults over the age of 40 with one chronic condition (39). He asked them to fill out a health assessment questionnaire, and based on the answers to this simple quiz, which consisted of largely behavior-related questions, the person was triaged to an appropriate risk group: diet, smoking, alcohol, exercise, and so forth. Pronk's paper revealed that this simple, straightforward, universally available information-providing strategy lowered health care costs per individual by an average of $2,000 a year. Distributed hypothetically across our population of about 300 million, this means $600 billion in potential savings, more than enough to hire thousands of health educators for our nation's schools.

Dee Edington of the University of Michigan provides data that indicate that one behavioral risk factor increases costs by 30% over the baseline, two by 70%, and so on, until seven risk factors lead to increased costs of 330%. It takes no imagination to develop the return on investment that attacking these modifiable risk factors would yield (40).

Similarly, in 1965, in their important Alameda, California, survey, Lester Breslow, professor of public health at UCLA, and his colleagues showed that those with no adverse health behaviors lived 30 years longer, on average, than those with five or more. In my mind many of the cost/benefit studies merely reflect different stages of fitness of the various populations (41).

My ideal program for Next Medicine begins with a health risk assessment for everyone, within the chosen HMO, perhaps every 5 years, using a wide variety of scientifically validated biomarkers. The life insurance industry has entire city blocks of accountants who know how to price premiums according to risk. On the health science side, we are rapidly generating rigorous predictive profiles that tell an individual or group with increasing accuracy what lies in their medical future. Poor health risk scores become luxury items requiring added expense. Good health risk scores are bargain items, "on sale."

I get help here from Steve Blair's critical *JAMA* article "Physical Fitness and All-cause Mortality," in which he and his colleagues analyzed data on thousands of individuals as a premium cost allocation tool (42). Young, fit females will live long and healthy lives and should pay less for their health insurance premium as a result. Conversely, older, unfit males with higher health risk and mortality rates will have premium costs that reflect their greater risk. Just as insurance companies "risk adjust" premium costs for teenage male drivers, so too will expanded health risk appraisal profiles provide rational tools that reflect the individual and collective burden on the resources of the Commonhealth. As we have seen, Blair uses measurement of $Vo_2$ max as his fitness biomarker. Other measurements—resting pulse rate, number of chair stands, half-mile completion time, and so forth—emerge as ancillary guides to higher or lower health care cost.

I predict that we will soon be able to get a gene profile on everyone by simply scraping the inside of their cheek with a cotton swab. This will provide the basis for a fitness profile that will predict future health outcomes with high precision. Less expense will be allocated to the fit gene profiles. To me, this is what the ballyhooed "personalized health" movement should represent, instead of what I perceive to be another covert strategy to feed the Big Pharma tiger. We must recognize that most biomarkers exhibit phenotypic plasticity—that is, they change for the better or worse according to lifestyle decisions. Therefore, this year's health insurance premium will be reduced in accord with next year's more fit gene profile resulting from improved lifestyle pursuit.

What remains, therefore, is to incentivize fitness through lower health insurance premiums. The more fit you are, the less you pay. The more disrespectful you are of your potential, the more you pay a logical risk adjustment. People in our society like the woman I encountered during my *Sonya Live* appearance need to pay more for neglecting their health, certainly not all at once, but over time. Eventually everyone needs to feel responsible for his or her own health and the cost of maintaining it. I believe in getting this group's attention through financial means to persuade them to take care of themselves and save us all a lot of money.

But I also know that I have the responsibility of helping her by providing more information and incentive to exploit her expanded self-efficacy. You and I, all of us share the responsibility of building every participant's personal responsibility for ensuring the Commonhealth. All citizens should participate in building a healthier nation. We have a collective cultural responsibility, not just an individual one.

We have now effectively defined health, measured it, and recognized its determinants. We have suggested how Next Medicine could be implemented. We have made real progress. Despite its recent vintage, the medical-industrial complex has put down major roots in the profits derived from illness. We must redeploy these profits so that repair medicine and preventive medicine are partners rather than competitors. Proposing a safety net of universal health coverage that is continually adjusting to demonstrated need does not preclude facelifts, boob jobs, and daily MRIs, if an individual is willing to pay for them. But I insist that such desires are not part of the Commonhealth. These individuals need to find a different commons on which to graze, and the polis is not going to pay for it.

I have pointed out repeatedly in this book that we have the good fortune to be living at the historic moment when the ignorance of fate has been replaced by the knowledge of choice, the tipping point, the inflection moment deeded to us by the new medical science of the past 50 years. For the very first time, we can confidently write the equation for health with rigorous coefficients and exponentials, which will constantly evolve and determine the operational details of Next Medicine. We have seen that Next Medicine uses information, education, opportunity, incentives, and disincentives to serve health needs at least as much as it serves illness needs. And we have seen that Next Medicine can be green. Now let's look at Next Medicine's influence on our communities and day-to-day lives.

# Healthier Communities

The problem with current medicine is the fundamental mismatch between its goals and its methods—between biology and capitalism. To resolve this mismatch we must examine the conflicting forces. Our biology, our nature, has been deeded to us by millions of years of ceaseless experimentation and produced us, a species that is very nearly perfect. Even if we have minor imperfections, we cannot re-engineer our nature. Capitalism, meanwhile, is the strategy we have chosen as the basis of our society's function. Since we have only recently created this structure, it is in our power to remake it. We need not deny capitalism's practical benefits; all we have to do is change the product it sells from disease to health. Why not?

At this climactic moment in American history, we are free to think anew, to challenge the old, and to enable the new. We relied on the medical market to offer a worthy product. It did not work. To make a categorical shift, it is clear that our national government must take a leading role. We need the federal government to oversee the structural reconfiguration of personnel, technology, education, and money. It must assume a major role in reshaping the ecology of medical care. But even acknowledging this, we must recognize that ultimately all change is local and personal.

So Next Medicine needs all of us, along with Washington. Theory must be matched by practice. Aristotle insisted that praxis was essential for democracy.

The will of the people must be made to work. "Of," "by," and "for" is not just a noble sentiment—it is a mandate. Next Medicine will emerge as we all take part.

## Together, We Can

Integral to the implementation of a full Commonhealth are the many American philanthropies, national and local. Of the many fine national foundations, the Robert Wood Johnson Foundation (RWJF) stands out. In 2008 it funded 1,000 grants in the amount of $520 million (1). Currently, it is putting up $66 million for Healthykids, a program addressing the 23 million American children and teenagers who are overweight. Our local group has submitted an application for a grant. RWJF emphasizes community-based solutions in its grant-making and is particularly concerned with the issue of a healthy environment.

More locally, community foundations play huge roles in assessing and addressing our needs. Because they are embedded in the community, they are able to lead the community to a better health platform. There are currently more than 650 community foundations nationwide, most of which have a direct or indirect commitment to health. Their efforts are in turn supported by thousands of others—service clubs, faith organizations, YMCA and YWCA, industry, and labor—each displaying a devotion to improved health individually and collectively. Together we can. Civitas regained.

Research psychologist Anita Stewart and I participated in her excellent program, Community Healthy Activity Model Program for Seniors (CHAMPS). Anita's group introduced physical activity in a dozen senior centers in the Bay area (2). Her contributions prevented many hip fractures, chased away depression, and saved Medicare millions of dollars, all through a coordinated, low-tech community effort.

Several years ago, I was invited to give the kickoff talk at the AARP headquarters in Washington for a new RWJF initiative, Blueprint for Activity, aimed at improving senior fitness. Numerous notable personages, including members of Congress, attended. The message of my talk was simple: "The grand value of physical exercise for all, but particularly for our older selves, is now securely established, proven, done with a red ribbon on it. Exercise is good, done. But how do you get people to do it?" That is the major unmet issue that looms even larger today than when I delivered my talk.

John Gardner insisted that all health is predominantly about community. "Common Cause" was a Gardner-inspired movement (3). In 1995, I wrote a white paper for him entitled "Health as a Community Asset." (4) The community as a locus for health is an emphasis of the Healthy People initiative promoted internationally by the World Health Organization and in America by the CDC. The Healthy People protocols provide advice to communities as they set up goals for achieving an improved health profile. Education is the emphasis, and the idea of Commonhealth is critical. The medical profession is important, but less so than involvement in community effort.

Intrinsic to the adoption of a community health perspective is the critical tactic known as "make the healthy choice the easy choice." Dr. Pekka Puska, director general of the Finnish National Public Health Service, has major experience in community health programs in North Karelia. He commented, "You can give people all kinds of information, but unless you make the healthy choice the easy choice it's not going to be the one that people make" (5). Parks, bike lanes, community gardens, farmers' markets, hosts of new community-driven intrinsic health protocols emerge. The RWJF has been an outspoken advocate for Active Living Communities (6). These communities have a specific town plan, and embedded in the general plan of the town, city, or county are zoning rules, ordinances, and other incentives that encourage the healthy, "easy choice." David Satcher, past director of the CDC, says that medical care *per se* does little to influence the determinant of health (7). What does? Shared partnerships, even including doctors. Ann Robertson of Toronto supplies the useful phrase, "moral economy of interdependence" (8).

If good food is a prime contributor to good health, but the neighborhood only has fast-food outlets, then you do not have a sound nutritional program. If the new health paradigm mandates adequate exercise, but there are no open spaces, parks, or safe biking/running paths, then knowing that exercise is valuable is worth nothing.

Several years ago, a group of Stanford medical students and I conducted an in-the-neighborhood assessment of the health needs of three ethnic groups— African-Americans, Hispanics, and Pacific Islanders—in East Palo Alto, California. We surveyed the groups on what health services they thought their neighborhood needed. The list we came up with was not surprising: more convenient clinics, after-hour services, a visiting nurse, a drugstore, and a convalescent home.

But what we received from the African-American group was astonishing. Their top priority was pit bull control. I was flabbergasted and expressed my shock to Roz Lasker, a noted health needs expert at the New York Academy of Medicine. She was totally sympathetic to their response: "If that is their perception, that is the reality," she said. So our group made recommendations to the appropriate authorities, and pit bull control was enforced, removing that impediment to taking a safe walk. Broken windows and graffiti similarly erode the chances for Commonhealth and Next Medicine. The Commonhealth enterprise needs the awareness and financing to address these less obvious but usually most substantive factors.

## Healthy Silicon Valley and Fit for Learning

As I phased out my medical practice in 2000, I welcomed the opportunity to do more at a community level. With John Gardner's help and blessings, a group of interested citizens organized into a group now known as Healthy Silicon Valley (HSV). We set out with an initial budget of $250,000, money obtained from seven local philanthropies. We nested HSV at the YMCA that serves as our administrative home. Our founding group hired a small staff and held a series of organizational meetings with a number of community groups. We debated priorities and eventually chose obesity as our first target, asserting the need for improved nutrition and physical activity.

A number of related protocols grew out of this early planning. The development I prize the most is the creation of what we call Fit for Learning, a grade-appropriate health curriculum with monthly themes that started with the cooperation and enthusiastic support of the supervisor of our County Board of Education. It is now in its fourth year, and the early results are exciting. This is an initiative that insisted that the schools should not stand passively by while a third of our schoolchildren become diabetic, as the CDC has predicted. Locally conceived and financed, our program involves every schoolchild in our county, about 250,000 of them. If a third of them were to become diabetic, this means that we would have 80,000 potential diabetes cases on our hands.

School cafeterias are stocked with calorically dense and nutritionally marginal fast food. Schools do not comply with the mandated physical activity curriculum. Although all states include a mandate for PE, only 13 include enforceable guidelines, and only 4 take any initiative to assure that schools comply. In this, my community is like most of America, but we wanted to do something about it—hence, Fit for Learning. We have more than 100 champions, lay cheerleaders for health-behavior change, in our schools, teachers and parents who help lead the children to better lifestyles. These champions in turn are augmented by the physician speakers' bureau that we are establishing.

We also have Youth Health Advocates, who have generated dozens of health-topic video public service announcements that are broadcast in the auditorium and recreation areas. One of my very favorite activities is talking to groups of grade-school kids. "I don't want to see you in my office or at Stanford Hospital with diabetes," I tell them. "I want you not to get diabetes in the first place." I feel that more good is being done by getting this message out than by all the endocrinologists and kidney dialysis providers in our area.

We are not alone. Kansas City recognized that 40% of its children are over-weight and has begun a Walk With Your Child program for parents. *Spark,* a recent book by Harvard's John Ratey (9), features the program in the Naperville school district outside Chicago. A small group of motivated citizens there was determined to say "no" to diabetes. They instigated a program called Fit4 Life, a close cousin of our own Fit for Learning. The children are given extensive material on how to stay healthy with nutrition and physical activity. Not coincidentally, the school's academic performance spurted and their attendance and behavioral pro-files improved. John Ratey is now on a crusade to sell the idea of brain fitness—the brain, after all, can be thought of as a muscle to which "use it or lose it" applies.

The coupling of academic and physical fitness brings to mind a wonderful visit that my father and I made to West Point 40 years ago. We addressed the best audience I have ever confronted—they hung on our every word. Their PE instructors were very proud to display a graph showing a direct correlation between class academic standing and physical test performance.

An article published in *USA Today* on June 15, 2009, and subsequently picked up by *Newsweek* featured the wonderful story of Albert Lea, Minnesota, a cozy small mid-Western town with health statistics like the rest: 40% over-weight, 30% hypertensive. The city manager and staff, seeking to pick up the town, applied for a "Vitality Project" grant from the sponsoring AARP. Because of the seeming commitment to action made in the application early in 2009, a four-pronged approach was instituted: (1) improving community environment (more gardens, bike lanes, farmers' markets, etc.), (2) creating social groups to exploit the new resources, (3) revamping home, work, and school habitats, and (4) building the inner self through motivational seminars. Twenty percent of the town's 18,000 residents took part (10,11). Early results of the study, which concluded in September 2009, show an average weight loss of 2.6 pounds, a projected increase in life expectancy of 3 years, and a 52% decrease in health care claims by city employees.

I hope that this and dozens of other far-flung grassroots efforts display a new viral reach to the Commonhealth, to a local of, by, and for the people ownership of their shared health.

## The Wider Community: The World

Singapore caught the school-age fitness bug in 1992. The people of this tiny country were alert enough to know that they could not sit by and wait for the epidemic of obesity to invade their school system. They began Trim and Fit (TAF), a series of interventions that we might consider draconian: refusing to promote students unless they achieve a certain weight loss goal, for instance.

A study from Denmark of 276,000 school-age children (tracked from 1930 to 1976) showed that heart disease in people in their 40s, 50s, and 60s was strongly correlated with their school-age weight (12). The study, reported in 2007, discovered that even when the overweight children lost weight as adults, they were still at greater risk for heart disease. The heavier the child, the greater the risk.

A couple of years ago, I took two trips to Cuba that provided me with unexpected insights. First, our group was informed that since the American embargo of basic goods such as gasoline and food, the Cuban incidence of obesity and diabetes had gone down, certainly contributing to their relatively healthy standing in the WHO survey (13). Maybe America should embargo itself. Later, we interviewed a number of Cuban medical students. As part of their fourth-year experience, they are obliged to practice Medicine up-country, in their own country and in neighboring Haiti and the Dominican Republic. They take their medical training into the countryside and experience the jolting realization that comes to every new medical student: how incompetent they are. Several of the students agreed that their most effective activity was working with the village priest, with whom they would meet the day before he delivered his Sunday sermon. The students would provide a basic health message for him to pass on to his faithful. As a result, handwashing, mosquito control, sound nutrition advice, and family planning were provided in a nontraditional medical fashion.

Borrowing from this powerful example, the Health Trust, a community organization dedicated to improving the health of Santa Clara County residents, has funded a group of local pastors and provided them with health messages for their parishioners, who have a very low health-literacy rate.

All these striking examples are part of the Commonhealth. The medical system is just one of the participating agencies in the Commonhealth, and usually the least important; self-efficacy and community responsibility are the more substantial determinants of health.

## The Lifelong Fitness Alliance

Thirty years ago, a group of like-minded Stanford runner friends founded the 50-Plus Runners Association. Initially it was informal and loose, a club based on a conviction that our shared exercise habit represented an opportunity to inform others that fitness was important in later life. I was an eager early member, since I had already run my first few Boston Marathons in my mid-40s and fully appreciated the euphoria that accompanies a fit lifestyle. Our first president, Peter Wood, is a British marathoner and an expert in cholesterol metabolism. Peter enlisted some of his running mates and discovered for the first time that running elevated the levels of the good HDL blood cholesterol (14). This small observation has been confirmed many times since and stands as an important data point in the literature about cholesterol and physical activity.

The mainstay of our first 10 years was Dr. Paul Spangler, who had been in my father's medical school class at Harvard. Spangler had consecrated his late years to championing the idea of senior fitness and to competing nationally in every Senior Games, in which he accumulated many gold medals. One day, in anticipation of his 5-mile run with us at our Stanford meeting, I asked him what he thought his time might be for the run. He replied, "I'm not sure, but whatever it is, it will be a world record." I hope I will be able to have the same perspective when I am in my mid-90s. He died in his 96th year while running in his hometown of San Luis Obispo, having failed in his avowed intent to be the first centenarian to run a marathon, but having succeeded brilliantly in showing us our potential.

Another of our stellar guests at the 50-Plus weekend was running legend Ron Clarke, who carried the Olympic torch for the 1980 Melbourne Olympics. In his remarks to our meeting, he recounted a race late in his career against the two great British runners Sebastian Coe and Steve Ovett. For the first three laps they competed evenly, but at the end the others prevailed, leaving Ron to come in third. He reflected, "The race of life goes not to the fastest starter but to the one who slows down last." This tortoise philosophy reassures me about my slowing life-pace. But I continue to run, content, hopefully, to finish last.

Jim Fries's research group at Stanford has chronicled the health experience of our membership (15). An article in a recent issue of the *Archives of Internal Medicine* covers 21 years of our membership (Fig. 13.1). Our disability and mortality are equivalent to those of an unfit community control group that is 20 or 30 years younger. Fitness is a major survival strategy. The fit should have lower health insurance rates instead of subsidizing those who sit.

We collaborated with the National Coalition for Promoting Physical Activity and the RWJF to assist Dr. David Chenowith in creating a physical inactivity cost calculator tool to assist groups interested in initiating exercise programs in their development (16).

## Fitness Ambassadors and Rx for Fitness

The two new programs of our renamed 50-Plus Lifelong Fitness Alliance are Fitness Ambassadors and the Rx for Fitness protocol. The ambassador program

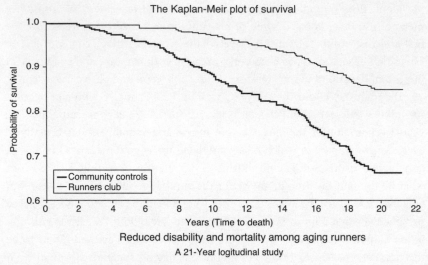

**Figure 13.1** Runners live longer better.

is a direct effort to spread the word of senior fitness. It rests on a strong theo-retical framework, based on two of Albert Bandura's steps for increased self-efficacy (17): step 2, peer examples; and step 3, social persuasion. Our fitness ambassadors encourage people to get from here to there on their own two legs.

Simply spreading health messages via print or other media, while necessary, will not generate much change in a community. Information delivery needs a catalyst to make the information sink in, and that catalyst is the ambassador. The ambassador is a personal mediating agent—a cheerleader and a champion (but a relevant champion).

To encourage an inactive person to become active, step 1 of Bandura's steps—small steps of mastery—is critical. Studies indicate that while getting an active person to become more active is always worthy, it is not as important as getting an inactive person to become a little more active. The first step is the most important, and the ambassador must be relevant to that first step. A mara-thoner has an additional burden in being an ambassador since inactive people are intimidated by others whom they do not see as being relevant to their place in life. Fundamentally, the ambassador is a volunteer who reaches out to stage walks, lectures, and social occasions, all with the intent of enlisting further recruits and saving Medicare's money.

To spread the word on a larger scale, we traveled to Washington to meet with Josefina Carbonel, then the Assistant Secretary of Aging in the Department of Health and Human Services, and present our ambassador program to her. The senior centers of America are supported by an ongoing congressional appropriation, the Older Americans Act. This mandates that every senior center have a nutrition counselor. That is a good start, but what about a fitness ambassador?

We continue to try to place fitness ambassadors into our local senior centers, and still hope to make the idea more widely adopted. But a Stanford colleague observed that not many older people actually visit senior centers; the one place that all older people do patronize is the doctor's office. Acknowledging this, we are developing an Rx for Fitness program. With the help of an electronic medical system, a physician who identifies a patient as in need of physical activity (virtually everybody) can simply check a box to generate a referral to the Lifelong Fitness Alliance office, and we will supply an ambassador for the patient.

We also made presentations to the AARP leadership about using our Fitness Ambassador program for their 33 million members. Their attention, however, seemed mostly taken up with their advocacy for the Medicare drug bill. We continue to romance each other with the idea that taking a walk is really more efficient and targeted than taking a pill.

These two locally generated programs, the Fitness Ambassador and the Rx for Fitness program, have cousins in hundreds of similar programs around the country, and represent a variety of other efforts to arrest the decline of frail elders, recognizing that as we age, our legs are our most important organs. These non-medical protocols offer great promise.

We have warehouses full of gene information, but almost nothing about health promotion and the community. The outstanding exception to this is the Stanford Five City Project led by my friend, medical epidemiologist Jack Farquhar (18). This involved five California cities—Salinas, Monterey, San Luis Obispo, Modesto, and Santa Monica—and 300,000 people overall. The object of the study was to determine whether a 20% reduction in cardiovascular disease could be achieved not by improving ambulance service or recruiting more cardiac surgeons, but by low-tech informational activities. The study targeted smoking and high blood pressure. It was supported by a large clinical trial grant from the NIH, and from Kaiser. Hundreds of articles have come out of the project. The results showed impressive drops in smoking and blood pressure, but one of the hoped-for results, a reduction in death rates, was not proven, as it was in the famous Karelia study in Finland (19). Using a similar protocol, the Finns were able to demonstrate a marked reduction in deaths from cardiovascular disease as a result of community interventions. Similar success was realized in Kerala, India, where a terribly impoverished community was able to come together and pursue a Commonhealth strategy. This is the model that needs to be replicated repeatedly.

The medical schools must also accommodate to a community approach. I have noted the ICU focus on the extreme right edge of the portrait of the ecology of medical care (see Fig. 4.1). Medical schools are fixated on this margin, remote from the community. Now numerous medical schools are guiltily seeking to address this inadequacy. Medical schools' products should match what the community needs, not what the academics proclaim the community needs—health, not disease, practitioners. The health-promotion curriculum demands parity with molecular biology.

The economic stimulus package would have done well to jumpstart these efforts to support and extend the CDC and our federal health promotion commitment with another $10 billion or so. But, more importantly, we should greatly expand the budgets of county health departments, which are closer to home and represent the community's health-promotion needs.

## Next Medicine: *Summa Logicae*

Next Medicine mandates that its structure support its mission of asserting and assuring human potential. Universal coverage born out of shared responsibility is close at hand. Mandatory insurance coverage in one of a series of comprehensive, integrated delivery systems run by a multi-representational board as a Commonhealth enterprise, like the Federal Reserve, will come to pass as political pressures demand a revolution. Heightened personal responsibility for healthy behavior will be abetted by information and incentives aligned in the pursuit of health.

Health care professionals of varied and new competencies will be salaried within the Commonhealth, with rewards for outstanding results measured by agreed-upon community performance standards. Prevention and maintenance efforts will achieve financial parity with repair. Health education in schools will be supported by generous monies made available thanks to prevention efforts. The community will have oversight of the budget.

Insurance coverage of all the uninsured and underinsured persons will be paid for by the hundreds of billions of dollars left over after we recapture the self-efficacy that had previously been deeded to the medical-industrial complex. Accidents and other unforeseeable, "nature's lottery," external-agency experiences will be covered by the basic insurance package, but expenses that occur due to lack of personal responsibility will be addressed by risk-adjustment costs.

Capitalism will support health instead of disease. America will more equitably distribute its riches to ensure the vitality of the Commonhealth through Next Medicine. Greatly expanded information technology will track the many delivery models that will quickly evolve.

Other countries' experiments, such as those in Holland and Australia, will help guide our efforts. The Dutch experience, based on the 2006 adoption of an Alain Enthoven "managed competition" model, is under intense international scrutiny (20). Holland has universal coverage, choice of provider, management oversight, and emphasis on primary care—all features of the ideal model. But like the Emanuel Fuchs proposal and others, it fails to mandate personal responsibility within its framework.

Unless and until people are required to commit to self-care and self-efficacy, any proposition is destined to fail. The health equation can be solved only with personal participation. Health must be owned and respected, not outsourced. The Commonhealth must be personal and common.

We must deal with the chilling recognition that our health may be deteriorating. An article in the Millbank Quarterly 2009, predicting shortening life expectancy, caught us all off guard (21). We had gotten so accustomed to decades of progressive life-lengthening reports that we serenely expected them to continue. But this cautionary article gave us great pause. And now we find that this projection was not just hypothetical, but astonishingly real. In April 2008, workers from Harvard and elsewhere surveyed the health and mortality statistics of more than 3,000 American counties (22). The death statistics spoke to the accuracy of the *NEJM* prediction: in 180 counties, life expectancy had shortened by 1.3 years.

A January 14, 2010, release on U.S. well-being by Gallup Healthways reports that five of six indices of well-being fell from 2008 to 2009. These indicators represent both subjective and objective measures of well-being. The message appears that despite our dollars spent and extravagant scientific know-how, we are doing worse on the things that matter most (23).

When we put this grim fact together with our children's obesity figures, we see that we are in for some bad times ahead. An August 19, 2008, report from the Trust for America's Health and the RWJF found that in the past year alone, obesity rates rose in 37 states. In 28 states, more than 25% of adults are obese. Only Colorado has obesity in less than 20% of its population (24).

Diabetes is the poster-child disease for the Next Medicine revolution, but the epidemic is much bigger than diabetes. It is more inclusively labeled the disuse syndrome, a collection of conditions that are inexorably destroying our potential. The fixes of Disease Medicine and Current Medicine, largely surgery and pills, do not work at all for the conditions of the disuse syndrome. There is no proxy for energy. You cannot buy, package, or invoke any alternative approach. But the heavy lifting in this instance is done by the individual and the society in which he or she lives.

Diabetes is an important test case for this claim. The Diabetes Prevention Trial of 2000 emphatically showed that modest lifestyle changes prevented most cases of diabetes, which are now at 20 million and rising. The survey paper, published in the *New England Journal of Medicine* (25), reported that 58% of the new diabetes cases can be prevented by less-than-vigorous physical exercise and diet, compared to 30% that are prevented by drugs. That 58%, in my mind, is minimal and could be virtually 100%. Diabetes shortens life expectancy by an average of 15 years per person. 600,000 times 15 years equals 9 million years of lost life potential because of a preventable disease to which Disease Medicine and Current Medicine are irrelevant. They find little room in their black bags for exercise, preferring pills and technology, because that is where the money is.

The benefits of physical exercise are established and many. There is a cascade of new papers addressing the Alzheimer's and Parkinson's disease pandemics, showing that physical fitness could relieve or retard them. I recall being astonished more than 20 years ago by Robert Dustman's paper on physical fitness and cognitive competence, published in the "obscure" journal *The Neurobiology of Aging* (26). It made me jump from my seat. For years, I had had to fend off multiple audience questions in the vein of "Is exercise good for the brain?" I had always deferred them, because we really had no data then. Dustman's early contribution has now been confirmed hundreds of times over, including via high-tech demonstrations with PET and CAT scans of the dynamic rewiring that exercise provides to the brain. So the brain/exercise axis is confirmed, with immense applications to the real world.

Dr. Robert Sallis, past president of the American College of Sports Medicine, has been leading a charge to get the medical-industrial complex to label exercise as medicine (27). I resist this label, because it conveys a clinical model. Pills and surgery are not in the standard Olympic athlete's regimen. "Take a walk, not a pill," is my mantra.

There are numerous strategies for successful aging in healthier communities. Prominent among these is regular attention to the sense organs of sight, hearing, and particularly balance. Poor balance can be addressed by the Flamingo Stand protocol (standing on one leg for 15 seconds or longer to help strengthen balance), which helps maintain the even keel vital to continued safe walking. Do not wait until 70% of your health reserve is spent before saving. The close connection between movement and survival is as true today as it was in the Serengeti era.

# Afterword

M y aim in writing this book was to draw on the deep wellsprings of my experience and distill from them the first principles on which a proposal for a new paradigm for Medicine, Next Medicine, might be based. The sites of the drilling extended from Stanford to Alice Springs, from the Mayo Clinic to Olduvai, from the NIH to Greensburg, Pennsylvania, from the Santa Fe Institute to the Borneo jungle, and from the Max Planck Institute to school assemblies in San Jose. The sampled wells were in offices, homes, laboratories, schools, rainforests, and corporate offices. Shamans and laureates helped in the drilling, but mostly my colleagues were the patients.

As René Dubos has written: "Medicine was, at the beginning of civilization, the mother of sciences, and played a large role in the integration of early cultures. Then it constituted for a long time a bridge over which science and humanism maintained some contact. Today it has once more the opportunity (breathtaking!) of becoming a catalytic force in civilization by pointing to the need and providing the leadership for the development of a science of man" (1).

In his stirring 1995 essay "National Renewal" John Gardner called upon the US to renew the high principles that prompted the creation of our nation (2). He amended the Declaration of Independence slightly: life, liberty and the pursuit of meaning. For John, for all of us, the meaning of America is codified in our founding principles, which provide the moral and intellectual guidance that assure every American the opportunity to achieve individual potential.

Medicine can claim the same high purpose. Medical Renewal as specified in Next Medicine is a similar call for nobility of virtue and practice.

The catalytic force of Next Medicine is designed to assert and assure our human potential, but its goal is not really new: the Oracle at Delphi pronounced that goal 2,500 years ago. It is time to reclaim the basic principles.

The recent meltdown in our financial system is a painful reminder of the heavy price we pay when we fail to keep a close eye on the events occurring on the commons. Vigilance requires that the medical system be exposed to strict review. We need capitalism to reconfigure its product for our benefit, rather than for our pain. Feeling worse and paying more is not a healthy prescription. We must return to the first principles from which all else derives.

When in the course of human events the people recognize that one of their most important institutions has veered from its mission and become a hazard, not only to its own integrity of purpose but to the overall Commonhealth, then a moral imperative arises, an absolute individual and collective responsibility to fix what has gone wrong. The new conceptual framework, the new paradigm is here (Fig. A.1). We must embrace it.

REPLACEMENT PARADIGM

| Current Medicine | Next Medicine |
|---|---|
| DISEASE | HEALTH |
| REPAIR | PREVENTION |
| EXTERNAL ... LOCUS of CONTROL ... INTERNAL | |
| STRUCTURE | FUNCTION |
| COMPONENT | SYSTEM |
| EPISODE | PROCESS |
| HIGH TECH | LOW TECH |
| SPECIALIST | PRIMARY CARE |
| FEE for SERVICE | PREPAY |
| PARTIAL .. INSURANCE COVERAGE .. UNIVERSAL | |
| RIGHTS | RESPONSIBILITY |
| BUSINESS | PROFESSION |

**Figure A.1** New paradigm.

Of the thousands of prescriptions that I have written in my life, of the thousands of patients I have tended, this is the most important prescription, for the most important patient, all of us.

If not now, when? If not here, where? If not we, who?

I here and now propose Next Medicine. We—individuals, the profession, and communities—will reform society and its institutions to serve health instead of disease.

Become who you are.

Know your health.

Live your health.

Live long. Seize potential, find flow.

Work long. The world needs you.

Be necessary, stay engaged.

Die short, nothing first, all at once, cheap, tame.

Leave worthy ripples.

# Notes

## Preface

1   Holmes OW. Quoted in Fabricant ND, ed. *Why We Became Physicians*. New York: Grune & Stratton, 1954.
2   Ethel Percy Andrus, formerly a high school principal in California, founded the National Retired Teachers Association (NRTA) in 1947 to provide health insurance coverage to retired teachers, and to all retirees in 1958. Andrus and Father got together to broaden the vision. Dad was well associated with the science leaders in aging at that time—Nathan Shock, Clive McCay, Alex Comfort, et al.—and with them was formulating the new view of healthy aging. The early alliance of Andrus, Bill Fitch, first director, and Dad was germinative of the AARP.
3   Bortz EL, Bortz WM. Major issues in aging. *GP* 1959;20:84–95.
4   Bortz WM. *Atherosclerosis*. Honors Thesis, 1951, Williams College, Williamstown, Mass.
5   Larsen NP. Atherosclerosis, an autopsy study. *Hawaii Med J* 1951;14:129–132.
6   Bortz EL. The hospital of the future. *The Modern Hospital* 1948 Special Issue Sept; 174–186.
7   Lynen F. Nobel Prize Acceptance Speech: *From Activated Acetic Acid to the Terpenes and Fatty Acids*. Stockholm, 12/11/1964.
8   Bortz EL. Geriatrics: a new interest for the doctor. *Medical World* 1940;58:219–221.
9   Cousins N. The anatomy of an illness (as perceived by the patient). *N Engl J Med* 1976;295:1458–1463.

10    Wallis V. *Two Old Women. An Alaskan Legend of Betrayal, Courage, and Survival*. New York: Harper Collins, 2004.

# Chapter 1

1    Siegler M. The progression from physician paternalism to patient autonomy to bureaucratic parsimony. *Archives of Internal Medicine* 1985;145:713–715.

2    Thomas L. *The Youngest Science*. New York: Viking Press, 1983.

3    Starr P. *The Social Transformation of American Medicine. The Rise of a Sovereign Profession and the Making of a Vast Industry*. New York: Basic Books, 1982.

4    Cousins NC. *The Physician in Literature*. Philadelphia: Saunders, 1982.

5    James W. *The Varieties of Religious Experience. A Study in Human Nature*. Originally published in 1902, reprinted in 1997 by Touchstone, New York.

6    Garibaldi M. Opinion: Matter of Farrell. New Jersey Supreme Court, 1987.

7    Reader WJ. *Professional Men: The Rise of the Professional Classes in 19th-Century England*. London: Weidenfeld and Nicholson, 1966.

8    Schlesinger M. A loss of faith: the source of reduced political legitimacy for the American medical profession. *Milbank Quarterly* 2002;80:1–45.

9    Kuhn T. *The Structure of Scientific Revolutions*. Chicago: University of Chicago Press, 1962.

10    Darwin C. *On the Origin of Species*. Cambridge: Cambridge University Press, 1859.

# Chapter 2

1    Aaron HJ, Schwartz WD. *The Painful Prescription: Rationing Hospital Care*. Washington, DC: Brookings Institute, 1984.

2    Morrison I. *Health Care in the New Millennium: Vision, Value, and Leadership*. San Francisco: Jossey-Bass, 2000.

3    Fogel R. *Health and Science*. International Longevity Center, Nov. 28, 2007.

4    WHO Health Report 2000: *Health Systems: Improving Performance*. Geneva: WHO.

5    Kaiser Family Foundation Health Care Marketplace, Feb. 8, 2006.

6    Starr P. *The Social Transformation of American Medicine: The Rise of a Sovereign Profession and the Making of a Vast Industry*. New York: Basic Books, 1982.

7    U.S. physicians' salaries provided by AlliedPhysicians.com, 2009.

8    Halvorson G, Isham GJ. *Epidemic of Care: A Call for Safer, Better, and More Accessible Health Care*. San Francisco: Jossey-Bass, 2003.

9    Milliman USA Healthcare Guidelines 2001. Claim Probability Distribution. Agency for Healthcare Research and Quality, 2002, Research Article #19.

10    Thinkprogress.org, Boomer Health Trends.com, Agency for Healthcare Research and Quality quarterly hospital diagnoses.

11  U.S. Bureau of Economic Analysis personal consumption expenditures, Tables, 2009.

12  Reinhardt U, Hussey PS, Anderson GF. US health care spending in an international context. *Health Affairs* 2004;23:10–25.

13  Cutler DM. *Your Money or Your Life. Strong Medicine for America's Health Care System*. New York: Oxford University Press, 2008.

14  Emanuel E, Fuchs VC. Who really pays for health care? The myth of personal responsibility. *JAMA* 2008;299:1057–1059.

15  Buffet W. Quoted in Thinkprogress.org, Dec. 8, 2009.

16  Jenny NW, Arbow E. Challenge for financing higher education. Rockefeller Institute Study, March 2004.

17  Meara ER, Richard S, Cutler D. The gap gets bigger: changes in mortality and life expectancy by education 1981–2000. *Health Affairs* 2008;27:350–360.

18  Woolf SH, Johnson RF, Phillips RL, et al. Giving everyone the health of the educated; an examination of whether social change would save more lives than medical advances. *Am J Public Health* 2007;97:675–683.

19  Boomerhealthtravel.com

20  McClellan M. Remarks at Stanford Medical School Health Policy Conference, June 5, 2009.

21  Volsky I. Wonkroom.thinkprogress.org, June 4, 2009.

22  Himmelstein DV, Thorne D, Warren E, Woolhandler S. Medical bankruptcy in the United States, 2007: Results of a national study. *Am J Med* 2009;122:741–746.

23  Selzer and Co. Dept. of Public Health Report 2005, Survey of Iowan Consumers. September 2005.

24  Martin Luther King Jr. Cited by Hillary Clinton at World Health Assembly May 14, 1995.

25  WHO Data and Statistics. Geneva: WHO, 2004.

26  World Bank Group. Beyond Economic Growth Report, 2009.

27  Elo IT, Preston SH. Effects of early life conditions on adult mortality: a review. *Population Index* 1992;58:186–212.

28  Smedley BD, Stith AY, Nelson AR, eds. *Unequal Treatment: Confronting Racial and Ethnic Disparities in Health Care*. Washington, DC: National Academies Press, 2002.

29  Gilmer TP, Kronick RG. Hard times and health insurance: how many Americans will be uninsured by 2010? *Health Affairs* 2009;28:573–577.

30  Marmot MG, Smith GD, Stansfield S, et al. Health inequalities among British civil servants: The Whitehall Study II. *Lancet* 1991;337:1387–1393.

31  Marmot MG. Employment grade and coronary heart disease in British civil servants. *J Epidemiol Commun Health* 1978;32:295–304.

32  Sapolsky R. Any kind of mother in a storm. *Nature Neurosci* 2009;12:1355–1356.

33  Juster RP, McEwen BS, Lupien S. Allostatic load as biomarker of chronic stress and impact on health and cognitive stress. *Neurosci Biobehav Rev* 2009 Oct 12 [E-pub].

34  Richter C. On the occurrence of sudden death. *Ann Psychosomatic Med* 1957;19:191–198.

35  Seligman MC, Rashid T, Parks AC. Positive psychotherapy. *Gen Psychol* 2006;8:774–788.

36  Fraga MT, Ballestar E, Pazstat MF. Epigenetics: differences arise during the lifetimes of monozygotic twins. *Proc Nat Acad Sci USA* 2005;102:10604–10609.

37  *The Electric Ben Franklin: A Quick Biography of Benjamin Franklin.* Available at: http://www.ushistory.org/franklin/info/index.htm

38  Daniels N. Just health and health are. *Am J Bioethics* 2001;1:3–15.

39  Daniels N. *Just Health Care.* New York: Cambridge University Press, 1985.

40  Newhouse JP. Medical costs and medical market: another view. *N Engl J Med* 1979;300:855–856.

41  Bloomfield D. Cited in Strauss M, ed. *Familiar Medical Quotations.* Boston: Little, Brown, 1968.

42  Half of what doctors know is wrong. *New York Times Magazine*, March 16, 2003.

43  How do you fix national health reform? Feb. 1, 2000 healthbeat.com.

44  Rochefort DA. Savoring the literature of medicine. *Health Affairs* 2004;23:284–285.

45  Lundberg G. Low-tech autopsies in the era of high-tech medicine. *JAMA* 1998;280:1273–1274.

46  Gilmer T, Schneiderman LJ, Teetzel H. The costs of nonbeneficial treatment in the intensive care setting. *Health Affairs* 2005;24:961–971.

47  Dorchin Y, Gopher D, Olsen M, et al. A look into the nature and causes of human error in the intensive care unit. *Critical Care Med* 1995;23:294–300.

48  Institute of Medicine. *To Err is Human: Building a Safe Health System.* Institute of Medicine Press, Dec. 1, 1999.

49  James JJ. Impacts of the medical malpractice slowdown in Los Angeles County: January 1976. *Am J Public Health* 1979 May;69(5):437–443.

50  Gertner J. Positive deviance: Eighth Annual Year of Ideas. *New York Times Magazine*, Dec. 14, 2008, p. 68.

51  Hirsch C, Sommers L, Olsen A. The natural history of functional morbidity in hospitalized older patients. *J Am Geriatrics Soc* 1990;38:1296–1303.

52  Berwick DM. What patient-centered should mean: confessions of an extremist. *Health Affairs* 2009;28:555–565.

53  Berwick DM, Calkins DR, Cannon M, et al. The 100,000 Lives campaign: setting a goal and a deadline for improving health care quality. *JAMA* 2006,295:324–327.

54  Kassirer J. *On the Take: How Medicine's Complicity with Big Business Can Damage Your Health.* New York: Oxford University Press, 2005.

55  Wilkes M, Dublin B, Shapiro M. Pharmaceutical advertisement in leading medical journals: expert assessment. *Ann Intern Med* 1992;166:912–919.

56  Stark P. CNN Morning News, Nov. 9, 1990.

57  Abelson R, Saul S. Ties to industry clouds a clinic's mission. *New York Times*, Dec. 12, 2005.

58  Krugman C. Increasing competition in the U.S. medical and pharmaceutical sectors. *New York Times*, Dec. 16, 2005.

59  Avorn J. Dangerous deception: hiding the evidence of adverse drug effects. *N Engl J Med* 2006;375:2169.

60  Armstrong D. How a famed hospital invests in devices it uses. *Wall Street Journal*, Dec. 12, 2005.

61  Angell M. Drug companies and doctors: a story of corruption. *New York Review of Books*, Jan. 15, 2009.

62  Pear R. Dead doctors report links dead doctors to payments by Medicare. *New York Times*, July 9, 2008.

63  Dash E. Former chief will forfeit $418 million. *New York Times*, Dec. 7, 2007.

64  Congressional Budget Office Report on Unnecessary Surgery, 1974.

65  Keeler EB. A model of demand for effective care. *J Health Econ* 1995;14:231–238.

66  Wright JG. Hidden barriers to improvement in the quality of care. *N Engl J Med* 2005;345:1612–1620.

67  Olshansky J, Hayflick L, Perls T. The hype and the reality. *J Geron A Biol Med Sci* June 2004;8:513–514.

68  Schoen C, Davis K, Howard S. National Scorecard on U.S. health system performance. Commonwealth Fund, July 07, 2008, vol. 1.

69  Komlos J, Breitfelder A. Are Americans shorter because they are fatter? A comparison of U.S. and Dutch children: height and BMI values. *Ann Human Biol* 2007;32:593–606.

70  de Beer H. Observations on the history of Dutch physical stature from the Late Middle Ages to the present. *Economics and Human Biology* 2004;2:45–55.

71  Ezzati AB, Friedman S, Kulkarni C, et al. Reversal of fortunes; trends in county mortality and cross-county mortality disparities in the United States. *PLoS Medicine*, April 22, 2008.

72  Wennberg J, Gittelson A. Small area variation in health care delivery. *Science* 1973;182:1102–1108.

73  Wennberg J, Freemann J, Culp W. Are hospital services reduced in New Haven or over-utilized in Boston? *Lancet* 1987;1:1185–1189.

74  Wennberg J. Practice variations and health care reform: connecting the dots. *Health Affairs* [E-pub Oct. 7, 2004].

75  Most influential policy maker of past 25 Years. *Health Affairs*, Nov. 1, 1997.

76  *Dartmouth Atlas*. Dartmouth Institute for Health Policy and Clinical Practice, 2007.

77  Wennberg J, Fisher E, Baker L, et al. Evaluating the efficiency of California providers in caring for patients with chronic illness. *Health Affairs* July–December 2005 [Web exclusive].

78  Dubois R, Brook R. Preventable deaths: who, how often, and why? *Ann Intern Med* 1988;109:582–589.

79  Evans R. Comments at Princeton Conference, 1998.

80  Best M. The growing challenge of diabesity. *NIH Medline Plus*, Winter 2008.

## Chapter 3

1  Gordon R. *The Alarming History of Medicine*. New York: St. Martin's Press, 1993.

2  Goodenough UW. *The Sacred Depths of Nature*. New York: Oxford University Press, 2008.

3  McKeown T. *The Origin of Human Disease*. Cambridge, MA: Basil Blackwell, 1988.

4  Haub C. World Population to Date. Population Reference Data Sheet, 1995.

5  Malthus T. *An Essay on the Principle of Population.* Originally published, 1798; Oxford University Classics, 2001.

6  Diamond J. *Guns, Germs, and Steel: The Fate of Human Societies.* London/New York: W.W. Norton, 1997.

7  De Maupertis, Principle of Least Action, 1756.

8  Wikipedia List of Famines. Accessed Dec. 20, 2009.

9  Klein R. *The Human Career: Human Biological and Cultural Origins.* Chicago: University of Chicago Press, 1989.

10  Trevathan W. *Evolutionary Medicine.* New York: Oxford University Press, 2004.

11  Obelisk of Rameses II. Egyptian Museum of Berlin.

12  Freud S. *The Complete Psychological Works of Sigmund Freud.* Edited and translated by J. Strachey, vol. 7. London: Hogarth Press.

13  Frank J. *Persuasion and Healing.* Baltimore: Johns Hopkins Press, 1961.

14  Cannon W. Voodoo death. *Am Anthropologist* 1942;44:169–189.

15  Conrad L, Wenn M, Nutter V, et al. *The Western Medical Tradition 800 BC–AD 1800.* Cambridge, UK: Cambridge University Press, 1992.

16  Sigerist HE. *A History of Medicine: Primitive and Archaic Medicine.* New York: Oxford University Press, 1955.

17  Porter R. *Greatest Benefit to Mankind: A Medical History of Humanity.* New York: W.W. Norton, 1990.

18  Osler W. *Sir William Osler: Aphorisms From his Bedside Teaching and Writing.* New York: Henry Schuman, 1950.

19  Tarnas R. *The Passion of the Western Mind: Understanding the Ideas that Have Shaped our World View.* New York: Crown Books, 1998.

20  Sigerist H. Asclepius and his cult. In: *A History of Medicine*, vol. 2. Oxford University Press, 1961.

21  DuBos R. Nature evolving. In Sobel E, ed. *Ways of Health.* New York: Harcourt Brace Jovanovich, 1979.

22  Raschke W. *The Archaeology of the Olympics and Other Festivities in Antiquity.* Madison: University of Wisconsin Press, 1957.

23  Longrigg JN. *Greek Rational Medicine.* London: Routledge, 1993.

24  Easton SC. *Roger Bacon and his Search for a Universal Science.* New York: Columbia University Press, 1952.

25  Harris S. *The End of Faith, Religion, Terror and the Future of Reason.* New York: W.W. Norton, 2007.

26  Meshberger FL. An interpretation of Michaelangelo's Creation of Adam based on neuroanatomy. *JAMA* 1990;264:1837–1844.

27  Boccacio G. *The Decameron.* Translated by M. Musa. New York: Signet Classics, 2002.

28  Haggard HW. *Devils, Drugs, and Doctors.* London: William Heinemann Books Ltd., 1929.

29  Leonardo drawings, North Wing Royal College of Windsor Castle, London, 1985.

30  Pare A. Wikipedia. Accessed Dec. 4, 2009.

31  Holmes OW. *Quotes and Images.* Project Gutenberg release #7545.

32  Ramsay M. *Professional and Popular Medicine in France 1770–1830.* New York: Cambridge University Press, 1988.

33  Robinson JO. The barber-surgeons of London. *Arch Surg* 1984;119:1171–1175.

34  *Benjamin Franklin Autobiography.* Mineola, NY: Dover, 1996.

35  *The Autobiography of Benjamin Rush: His Travels Through Life Together with the Commonplace Book for 1789–1813.* Greenwood Press Reprint.

36  Derham J. *First 3 African American Physicians.* Available at: http://www.essortment.com/all/africanamerican_rqdo.htm

37  The Death of George Washington 1799. Available at: http://www.eyewitnesstohistory.com/washington.htm.

38  Rutkow I. *Bleeding Blue and Gray: Civil War Surgery and the Evolution of American Medicine.* New York: Random House, 2005.

39  Hardy A. *The Epidemic Streets: Infectious Disease and the Rise of Preventive Medicine.* New York: Oxford University Press, 1993.

40  Gelson GL. *The Private Science of Louis Pasteur.* Princeton: Princeton University Press, 1995.

41  Bernard C. *An Introduction to the Study of Experimental Medicine.* 1865. Translated by H.G. Green, 1927.

42  Cannon W. *The Wisdom of the Body.* New York: Norton Library, 1932.

43  F.G. Banting, co-discoverer of insulin. *JAMA* 1966;198:660–661.

44  Allen FL. New Medical Institute Jersey Institute for Diabetes and Metabolic Disorders. Open Discovery *New York Times*, April 27, 1921.

45  Joslin EP. Abolishing diabetic coma. *JAMA* 1929;93:33–40.

46  Medicine: Protosil. *Time Magazine,* Dec. 28, 1936.

47  MacFarlane G. *Alexander Fleming, The Man and the Myth.* New York: Oxford University Press, 1985.

48  Watson J. *The Double Helix: A Personal Memoir of the Structure of DNA.* Athenaeum, 1968.

49  Arthur Kornberg's remarks at Stanford Human Genome celebration.

50  Annual Report of the President of Harvard College, 1870–1871.

51  Beecher HW, Altschule M. *Medicine at Harvard :The First Three Hundred Years.* Hanover, NH: University Press of New England, 1977.

52  The Free Library by Farlex, July 1, 2009.

53  Flexner A. Medical Education in the United States and Canada, Bulletin no. 4. New York: Carnegie Foundation for the Advancement of Teaching, 1910.

54  Kett J. *The Formation of the American Medical Profession.* New Haven: Yale University Press, 1968.

55  Fishbein M. History of the American Medical Association. Special Article, Chapter 5: The First Annual Session. *JAMA* 1946;132:852–854.

56  Millenson M. *Demanding Medical Excellence.* Chicago: University of Chicago Press, 1997.

57  Kelley BM. *Yale: A History.* New Haven: Yale University Press, 1974.

58  Clapesattle H. *The Doctors Mayo.* Minneapolis: University of Minnesota Press, 1968.

59  Starr P. *The Social Transformation of American Medicine*. New York: Basic Books, 1984.

60  Bush V. Report of the Medical Advisory Committee Science: The Endless Frontier. 1945. National Science Foundation reprint Washington, DC, 1960.

61  Conference Proceedings, The Dynamic and Energetic Basis of Health and Aging, November 2002, NIH, Bethesda, Md.

## Chapter 4

1   Porter R. *The Greatest Benefit to Mankind: A Medical History of Humanity*. New York: W.W. Norton, 1990.

2   Voltaire, quoted in Strauss WM, ed. *Familiar Medical Quotations*. Boston: Little Brown, 1968.

3   Brenner BJ, Hall CJ. Computed tomography: an increasing source of radiation exposure. N Engl J Med 2007;357:2277–2284.

4   Kramer B. Cancer screening: a special clash of medical science and intuition. Lecture, NIH Clinical Center, Nov. 25, 2008.

5   Halvorson G, Isham G. *Epidemic of Care: A Call for Better and More Accountable Health Care*. New York: Wiley, 2003.

6   Kohane I. The incidentalome: a threat to genomic medicine. *JAMA* 2006;296: 212–215.

7   Herodotus. *Histories II 84*, translated by William Beloe.

8   Relman A. Medical industrial complex. *N Engl J Med* 1980;303:963–969.

9   Starr P. *The Social Transformation of American Medicine*. 1982 Basic books, New York Harvard Univ Press Cambridge Mass

10  Osler W. *Sir William Osler: Aphorisms From his Bedside Teaching and Writing*. New York: Henry Schuman, 1950.

11  *Aphorisms of Dr. Charles Horace Mayo and Dr. William James Mayo*. Springfield, Ill.: Charles Thomas, 1951.

12  Debley T, Stewart J. *The Story of Dr. Sidney R. Garfield: The Visionary Who Turned Sick Care into Health Care*. Portland, Oregon: Permanente Press, 2009.

13  Enthoven AC. Consumer choice health plan. Inflation and inequity in health care today with alternatives for cost control and an analysis of proposals for national health insurance. *N Engl J Med* 1978;288:650–658.

14  White KL, Williams TF, Greenberg BG. The ecology of medical care. *N Engl J Med* 1961;265:885–892.

15  Green LA, Fryer GE, Yawn BP. The ecology of medical care revisited. *N Engl J Med* 2001;344:2021–2025.

16  Christensen C, Grossman J, Hwang J. *The Innovative Prescription; A Disruptive Solution for Health Care*. New York: McGraw, 2009.

17  Leigh B, Kravitz R, Schembri M. Physician career satisfaction across specialties. *Arch Intern Med* 2002;162:1577–1584.

18   Scheurer D, McKean S, Miller J, et al. U.S. physician satisfaction: a systematic review. *J Hosp Med* 2009;4:560–566.

19   Haggerty R. Effectiveness of Medical Care. *NEJM* 1973;289:372–373.

20   Scrimshaw NS, Arroyave G, Bressau R. Nutrition. *Ann Rev Biochem* 1958;27: 403–436.

21   McDermott WK, Deuschle W, Barnett CR. Health care experiment at Many Farms. Science 1972;175:23–31.

22   Goodrich CH. Olendzki M, Deuschle KW Mt. Sinai;s Approach to the E. Harlem Community. *Bull. NY Acad. Med* 1970;41:97–112.

23   Annas G. Quoted by Lamm R in *Brave New World of Health Care.* Golden, Colorado: Fulcrum Press, 2003.

## Chapter 5

1   Bell D. *The Cultural Contradictions of Capitalism.* New York: Basic Books, 1976.

2   Riley MW, et al. *Age and Structural Lag.* New York: Wiley, 1994.

3   O'Dea K. Marked improvement in carbohydrate and lipid metabolism in Australian aborigines after temporary revision to traditional lifestyle. *Diabetes* 1984;33:596–603.

4   *Dartmouth Atlas of Health Care.* Dartmouth Institute for Health Policy and Clinical Practice, Lebanon, NH, 2010.

5   Grove A. Efficiency in the health care industries: a view from outside. *JAMA* 2005;294:490–492.

6   Woolhandler S, Campbell S, Himelstein D. Costs of health care administration in the United States and Canada. *N Engl J Med* 2005;349:768–773.

7   Bartlett D, Steele J. *Critical Condition: How Health Care in America became Big Business and Bad Medicine.* New York: Random House, 2004.

8   Gadamer HG (translated by Gangier J, Walker N). *The Enigma of Health: The Art of Healing in a Scientific Age.* Stanford, Calif.: Stanford University Press, 1996.

9   Illich I. *Limits to Medicine: Medical Nemesis, The Expropriation of Health.* New York: Marion Boyars, 1975.

10   Bortz, W. Reinventing Health Care From Panacea to Hygeia 2010 State of the World Transforming Cultures WW Norton, 2010 NY London.

## Chapter 6

1   Jefferson T, et al. The Declaration of Independence.

2   James W. Quoted in www.famousquotesandauthors.com.

3   Kuhn T. *The Structure of Scientific Revolutions.* Chicago: University of Chicago Press, 1962.

4   Plato. *The Republic.*

5   Verghese A. The Myth of Prevention. *Wall Street Journal,* June 20, 2009.

6   Obama B. Talk to House of Delegates AMA, June 15, 2009, Chicago. www. huffingtonpost.com.

7   Precope J. *Hippocrates on Diet and Hygiene.* London: Williams, Lea and Co.

8   McGinnis JM, Foege W. Actual causes of death. *JAMA* 1993;270:2207–2212.

9   Schroeder S, Shattuck Lecture *We can do Better Improving the Health of the American People* NEJM 2007;357:1221–1228.

10  Dubos R. Hippocrates in modern dress. In Sobel D, ed. *Ways of Health.* New York/London: Harcourt Brace Jovanovich, 1979.

11  Deming WE. Wikipedia. Accessed December 29, 2009.

12  Bandura A. *Self-Efficacy: The Exercise of Self-Control.* New York: Freeman, 2001.

13  Gardner J. National Renewal Independent Sector, National Civic League, 1995.

14  Knowles J. The balanced biology of the teaching hospital. In *Hospitals Doctors, and the Public Interest.* Cambridge, Mass.: Harvard University Press, 1955.

15  Seligman M. *Helplessness: On Depression, Development, and Death.* San Francisco: W.H. Freeman, 1975.

16  Lorig K, Ritter P, Dost A, et al. The Expert Patients Program on-line:1 year of an internet based self-management programme for patients with long-term conditions. *Chronic Illness* 2008;4:247–256.

17  Knowles J. The responsibility of the individual in doing better and feeling worse. In Knowles J, ed. *Health in the United States.* New York: W.W. Norton, 1977.

18  Fuchs V. *Who Shall Live? Health, Economics, and Social Choice.* Singapore: World Scientific, 1998.

19  Blank R. *The Price of Life: The Future of American Health Care.* New York: Columbia University Press, 1997.

20  Daniels N. Personal communication.

21  Emanuel E, Fuchs V. Who really pays for health care? The myth of shared responsibility. *N Engl J Med* 2008;299:157–159.

## Chapter 7

1   Aristotle. *Nichomachean Ethics.* Oxford World Classics, 1980.

2   Albert Einstein quotes: http://rescomp.stanford.edu/~cheshire/EinsteinQuotes.html

3   Anderson PM. More is different. *Science* 1972;177:393–396.

4   Morowitz H. *The Emergence of Everything: How the World Became Complex.* New York: Oxford University Press, 2002.

5   Pope John Paul II. *Fides et Ratio.* Papal Encyclical, Rome, 8/14/98.

6   Dawkins R. *The Selfish Gene.* New York: Oxford University Press, 1976.

7   Durham WL. *Co-Evolution: Genes, Culture, and Human Diversity.* Stanford, California: Stanford University Press, 1977.

8   Ho MW. *The Rainbow and the Worm: The Physics of Organisms.* Singapore: World Scientific, 1998.

9   Schrodinger E. *What Is Life? The Physical Aspects of Living Cells.* Cambridge, UK: Cambridge University Press, 1967.

10  Snow CP. *The Two Cultures and the Scientific Revolution* Cambridge, UK: Cambridge University Press, 1959.

11  Prigogine I, Stengers I. *Order Out of Chaos.* New York: Bantam, 1984.

12  Wicken J. *Evolution, Thermodynamics and Information: Extending the Darwinian Paradigm.* New York: Oxford University Press, 1987.

13  Corning P. *Nature's Magic Synergy in Evolution and the Fate of Mankind.* Cambridge, UK: Cambridge University Press, 2005.

14  Schneider E, Sagan D. *Into the Cool Energy Flow, Thermodynamics and Life.* Chicago: University of Chicago Press, 2005.

15  Weinberg S, quoted by Davidoff N, The Civil Heretic, *New York Times Magazine,* March 3, 2009.

16  Dyson F. *Origins of Life.* Cambridge, UK: Cambridge University Press, 1999.

17  Von Neumann J. Wikipedia, accessed January 7, 2010.

18  Darwin C. *Origin of Species.* Cambridge, UK: Cambridge University Press.

19  Koshland D. The seven pillars of life. *Science* 2002;295:2215–2216.

20  Veech RL. Personal communication.

21  Bernard C. *An Introduction to the Study of Experimental Medicine.* Originally published 1865. Translated by Green HG, 1927.

22  Cannon W. *The Wisdom of the Body.* New York: WW Norton, 1932.

23  Yates FE. Homeokinetics/homeodynamics: a physical heuristic for life and complexity. *Ecological Psychology* 2008;20:148–179.

24  Bortz WM. The physics of frailty. *J Am Geriatrics Soc* 1993;41:1004–1008.

25  McKeown T. *The Origins of Human Disease.* Oxford, UK: Basil Blackwell, 1988.

26  West Eberhard MT. *Developmental Plasticity.* New York: Oxford University Press, 2007.

27  Braam J, Davis R. Rain-, wind-, and touch-induced expression of calmodulin and calmodulin-related genes in Arabadopsis. *Cell* 1990;60:357–364.

28  Secor S, Fehsenfeld P, Diamond J. Responses of python gastrointestinal regulatory peptides to feeding. *Proc Natl Acad Sci USA* 2001;98:1367–1342.

29  Wolff J. Das Gesetz der Trannsformation der Knocken. Kirschwald, 1899; translated by Maquet P, Furlong R. Berlin: Springer Verlag, 1986.

30  Carter DM,Wong M, Orr T. Musculoskeletal autogeny, phylogeny and functional adaptation. *J Bi omech* 1991 (supp):3–16.

31  Fuller B. Tensegrity. *Portfolio and Art News Annual,* 1961.

32  Currens J, White PD. Half a century of running: clinical, psychologic and autopsy findings in the case of Clarence DeMar (Mr. Marathon). *N Engl J Med* 1961;265: 988–995.

33  Haskell WL, Sims C, Bortz WM, et al. Coronary artery size and dilating capacity in ultradistance runners. *Circulation* 1993;87:1076–1082.

34  Diamond M. Extensive cortical depth measurements and neuron size increase in the cortex of experimentally enriched rats. *J Comp Neurol* 1967;131:357–364.

35  Diamond M, Hopson J. *Magic Trees of the Mind: How to Nurture your Child's Intelligence, Creativity, and Healthy Emotions from Birth until Adolescence.* New York: Dutton, 1998.

36   Falk D. In Baltes Blog.com, April 18, 2009.

37   Treffert D, Chambers D. Inside the mind of a savant. *Scientific American*, June 2006.

38   Singh JAL, Zingg RM. *Wolf Children and Feral Man*. Denver: Archon Books, 1966.

39   Diamond J. Evolution of biologic safety factors. In: Weibel E, Taylor R, Bolis L, eds. *Principles of Animal Design*. Cambridge, Mass: Cambridge University Press, 1998.

40   Weibel ER. *Symmorphosis: On Form and Function in Shaping Life*. Cambridge, Mass.: Harvard University Press, 2000.

41   Heraclitus. Internet Encyclopedia of Philosophy. Available at: www.iep.utm.edu/

42   Spalding KL, Bhardwal RD, Bucholz D, et al. Retrospective birth dating of cells in humans. *Cell* 2005;122:4–6.

43   Sagan D. In Margulis L, Sagan D. *What is Life?* New York: Simon & Schuster, 1995.

## Chapter 8

1    Sheehan G. *Running and Being: The Total Experience* Red Bank, NJ: Second Wind, 1979.

2    Sheehan G. *Going the Distance: One Man's Journey to the End of His Life*. New York: Villard, 1996.

3    Margulis L, Sagan D. *What Is Life?* New York: Simon & Schuster, 1995.

4    U.S. Department of Health & Human Services. *Healthy People 2010; Understanding and Improving Health*. Washington DC, 2001.

5    World Health Organization, Ottawa Charter International Conference on Health Promotion. Nov. 21, 1986, Ottawa, Canada.

6    Szent Gyorgy remarks.

7    Precope J. *Hippocrates on Diet and Hygiene*. London: Zeno, n.d.

8    Kant I. *Critique of Pure Reason* (originally published 1781). London: Penguin Classics, 2007.

9    Maslow AH. A theory of human motivation. *Psychology Reviews* 1943;50:370–396.

10   Brabazon J. *Albert Schweitzer: A Biography*. New York: GP Putnam, 1975.

11   Gadamer HG. *The Enigma of Health: The Art of Healing in a Scientific Age*. Stanford, Calif.: Stanford University Press, 1996.

12   Illich I. *Limits to Medicine: Medical Nemesis: The Expropriation of Health*. London/ New York: Marion Boyars, 1995.

13   Dubos R. Hippocrates in modern dress. In: Sobel D, ed. *Ways of Health: Holistic Approaches to Ancient and Contemporary Medicine*. New York/London: Harcourt, Brace Jovanovich, 1979.

14   STEPS Center. Sole RV Goodwin BC. Signs of Life. How Complexity Pervades Biology Basic Books 2000 New York 2007.

15   Stanford Encyclopedia of Philosophy, Goodwin BC. The Life of Form Emergent Patterns of Morphological Transformations C R Acad Sci III 2000;373:15–21.

16   Stanford Knowledgebase. Lutz J. Flow and Sense of Coherence Two Aspects of the Same Dynamic? Global Health Proc. 2009;16:63–67.

17    Schuldberg D. Theoretical Contribution of Complex Systems to Positive Psychology and Health; A Somewhat Complicated Affair 2002. *Non Linear Dynamics, Psychology and Life Sciences.* 6:335–350.

18    Wilensky U. Emergent Entities and Emergent Processes: Constructing Emergence Through Multi-Agent Processing. Paper Presented at Conference American Educational Association, 2001.

19    Herophilus, quoted in Sextus Empiricus in Adversus Ethicus XJ 50. http://worldofquotes 1/7/2004.

20    Hippocrates. *A Regimen for Health,* quoted famousquotessite.com 9. Trans. Chadwick, Mann.

21    Plato. Newworldencyclopedia.com.

22    Huang-di. *The Yellow Emperor' Classic of Internal Medicine.* Translated by J. Veith *in Other Ways of Health* cited above.

23    Descartes R. *Discours de la Methode,* Pt. VI. Translated by J. Veith.

24    Disraeli speech, June 23, 1877. In: *Familiar Medical Quotations.* Boston: Little, Brown,

24A   CICERO de Legibus Book 3 Loeb Classical Library Harvard, 1968.

25    Dawkins R. *Unweaving the Rainbow: Science, Delusion and the Appetite for Wonder.* New York: Houghton Mifflin, 1998.

26    Gleick J. *Isaac Newton.* New York: Vintage Books, 2004.

27    Pendergast DR, Fisher NM, Calkins E. Cardiovascular, neuromuscular and metabolic alterations with age leading to frailty. *J Geron Biol Sci Med Sci* 1993; 48(Special Issue I):61–67.

28    Verdery R. Failure to thrive. In: Hazzard RR, Bierman E, Blass J, et al. *Principles of Geriatric Medicine and Gerontology.* New York: McGraw Hill, 2003.

29    Diamond J. Evaluation of biological safety factors: a cost/benefit analysis. In: Weibel ER, Taylor CB, Bolis L, eds. *Principles of Animal Design.* Cambridge, Mass.: Cambridge University Press, 1998.

30    Biewener A. Biomechanics and mammalian locomotion. *Science* 1990;250: 1205–1211.

31    Leaf A. Every day's a gift when you are over 100. *National Geographic* 1973;143:92–119.

32    Allard M, Robine JM. *Les Centenaires Francais.* Etude de la Fondation IPSEN L'Annee Gerontologique Supp. Paris, 2000.

33    Los Angeles Gerontology Research Group (www.grg.org).

34    Hulbert AJ, Camplon RP, Buffenstein R. Life and death, metabolic rate, membrane composition, and lifespan. *Physiol Rev* 2007;87:1175–1213.

35    Rubner M. *Das Problem des Lebensdauer.* Munich: Oldenborg, 1908.

36    Pearl R. *The Rate of Living: Being an Account of Some Experimental Studies in the Biology of Life Duration.* New York: Knopf, 1928.

37    Gould S. *The Panda's Thumb.* New York: WW Norton, 1980.

38    McCay CM, Maynard LA, Sperling G, et al. Effect of retarded growth upon the length of lifespan and the ultimate body size. *J Nutrition* 1935;10:63–74.

39    Harman DA. Aging: a theory based on free radical and radiation chemistry. *J Geron* 1956;11:293–312.

40    Denvir MA, Gray GA. Run for your life: exercise, oxidative stress and the aging endothelium. *J Physiol* 2009;587:4137–4138.

41  Sohal BS, Sohal BH, Orr WC. Mitochondrial superoxide and hydrogen peroxide generation, protein oxidative damage and longevity in different species of flies. *Free Radical Biol Med* 1995;19:499–504.

42  Manton K. Changing concepts of morbidity and mortality in the elderly population. *Milbank Memorial Fund Quarterly* 1982;60:183–244.

43  Giles J. Scientific wagers: wanna bet? *Nature* 2002;420:351–354.

44  Olshansky SJ, Passaro DJ, Hersher RC, et al. A potential decline in life expectancy. *N Engl J Med* 2005;352:1138–1142.

45  Finch CE. Evolution of the human lifespan and diseases of aging: roles of infection, inflammation, and nutrition. *Proc Natl Acad Sci USA* Dec. 4, 2009 [epub].

46  UNICEF. *Tracking Progress in Child and Maternal Nutrition: A Survival and Development Priority,* 2009.

47  Bortz WM, Bortz WM. How fast do we age? *J Geron A Biol Sci Med Sci* 1996;51A:M223–225.

48  Sehl M, Yates FE. Kinetics of human aging, I: rates of senescence between ages 30 and 70 in healthy persons. *J Geron B Biol Sci Med Sci* 2001;56B:198–208.

49  Sehl M, Pincus SM, Yates FE. Rates of senescence between ages 30 and 70 years in healthy people[pe: a questionnaire model predicting a non-linear an increasing risk of frailty and mortality (submitted).

50  Iglehart JK. Influences on the health of the population. *Health Affairs* 2002; 21:7–8.

51  Bortz WM. Biologic determinants of health. *Am J Pub Health* 2005;95:389–392.

52  Yates FE. Modeling frailty: can a simple feedback model suffice? *Mech Aging Devel* 2008;129:671–672.

53  Lewontin R, Rose S, Kamin L. *Not in Our Genes: Biology, Ideology and Human Values.* New York: Pantheon Books, 1984.

54  West-Eberhard MJ. *Developmental Plasticity.* New York: Oxford University Press, 2007.

55  Dawkins R. *The Selfish Gene.* New York: Oxford University Press, 1976.

56  McClintock B. In: Moore JA, ed. *The Discovery and Characterization of Transposable Elements: The Collected Papers of Barbara McClintock.* Garland, 1987.

57  Strohman R. Ancient genomes, wise bodies, and unhealthy people; limitations of a genetic paradigm in biology and medicine. *Perspec Biol Med* 1983;37:112–145.

58  Feinberg AP. Epigenetics at the epicenter of modern medicine. *JAMA* 2008;299: 1345–1350.

59  Tanner CM, Goldman SM, Landston WC, et al. Parkinson's disease in twins: an etiologic study. *JAMA* 1999;281:341–346.

60  Zaretsky M. Communication among fraternal twins; health behavior and social factors are associated with longevity that is greater among identical than fraternal U.S. World War II veteran twins. *J Geron Biol Sci Med Sci* 2003;58:566–572.

61  Pasteur L. In: Gelson GL. *The Private Science of Louis Pasteur.* Princeton University Press, 1995.

62  Holmes OW. Songs in Many Keys for the Meeting of the National Sanitary Association, 1866. In: *Familiar Medical Quotations.* Boston, Little Brown.

63  Prigogine I, Stengers I. *Order Out of Chaos.* New York: Bantam, 1984.

64  Ferringo R. Tour de France History: The World's Greatest Cycling Event. Doc's Sports Service 6/29/05.

65  Kasch FW, Boyer JL, Van Camp S, et al. Cardiovascular changes with age and exercise. *Scand J Sci Sports* 1995;5:147–151.

66  WHO Child Info. Monitoring the Situation of Children and Women. Available at: www.childinfo.org

67  Newman C. The heavy cost of fat. *National Geographic* August 2004.

68  Bortz W. Metabolic consequence of obesity. *Ann Intern Med* 1969;71:833–843.

69  Selye H. *The Story of the Adaptation Syndrome.* Montreal: Acta, 1952.

70  McEwen BS. Allostasis, allostatic load and the aging nervous system: role of excitatory amino acids and excititoxicity. *Neurochem Res* 2001;25:1219–1231.

71  Seeman TE, Singer BH, Rowe JW, et al. Price of adaptation: price of allostatic load and its health consequences. *Arch Intern Med* 1997;157:2259–2268.

72  Bortz W. The disuse syndrome. *West J Med* 1984;141:691–694.

73  Kraus H, Raab W. *Hypokinetic Disease: Disease Produced by the Lack of Exercise.* Springfield, Ill.: Charles C. Thomas, 1961.

74  Booth F. Sedentary death syndrome. *Am J Appl Physiol* 2004;29;447–460.

75  Lakdawalla D, Philipson T. The growth of obesity and technologic change. *Econ Human Biol* Epub Oct. 29, 2009:283–293.

76  Robinson TN. Television viewing and pediatric obesity. *Pediatr Clin North Am* 2001;48:1017–1023.

77  Santa Clara County Department of Health statistics.

78  Levine JA. Non-exercise activity thermogenesis. *Nutrition Rev* 2004;62s:82–97.

79  CDC MMR 2009.

80  Prentice AM, Jebb SA. Obesity: gluttony or sloth? *Br Med J* 1995;437–439.

81  Blair S. Surgeon General Report on Physical Activity and Health. *CDC*, 1996.

82  Blair SN, Kohl HW, Paffenbarger RS, et al. Physical fitness and all-cause mortality; a prospective study of healthy men and women. *JAMA* 1989;262:2395–2401.

83  Sui X, La Monte MJ, Laditka JN, et al. Cardiorespiratory fitness and adiposity as mortality predictors in older adults. *JAMA* 2007;298:2507–2516.

84  Fiatarone M, Marks E, Ryan N, Evans W. Strength training in nonagenarians. *JAMA* 1990;63:3029–3034.

85  Kaufman FR. *Diabesity.* New York: Random House, 2005.

86  Stampfer MJ, Colditz GA, Willett WC. A prospective study of moderate alcohol drinking and risk of diabetes in women. *Am J Epidemiol* 1998;128:549–558.

87  Manson JE, Ajani UA, Liu AS, et al. A prospective study of cigarette smoking and the incidence of diabetes mellitus among U.S. male physicians. *Am J Med* 2000;109: 538–547.

88  Finley LD, La Monte CE, Waslien CI, et al. Cardiorespiratory fitness, macronutrient intake and the metabolic syndrome. *J Am Dietetic Assoc* 2006;106:673–685.

89  Erikson K, Lindgrade F. Prevention of type II diabetes by diet and exercise. *Diabetologia* 1991;34:891–898.

90  Di Francesco-Marino S, Sciartelli A, DiValerio V. The effect of physical exercise on endothelial function. *Sports Med* 2009;39:787–812.

91    Carrell A. *Man the Unknown*. New York/London: Harper Bros., 1935.

92    Hayflick L. Aging under glass. In: Maramorosh K, ed. *Advances in Cell Culture*. Orlando: Academic Press, 1988.

93    Shock N. Mortality and measurement of aging. In: Strehler B, ed. *Biology of Aging*. Washington DC: American Institute of Biological Sciences, 1960.

94    Hayflick L. Biological aging is no longer an unsolved problem. *Ann NY Acad Sci* 2007;1100:1–13.

95    DeVries H, Wiswell W, Romero G, et al. Comparison of oxygen effects in young and old subjects. *Eur J Applied Physiol Occup Physiol* 1982;49:277–286.

96    Bortz W. Redefining human aging. *J Am Geriatrics Soc* 1987;37:1092–1096.

97    Aaron HJ, Schwartz WB, eds. *Coping with Methuselah: The Impact of Biology on Medicine and Society*. Washington, DC: Brookings Institution Press, 2004.

98    Rowe J, Kahn R. Human aging; usual and successful. *Science* 1987;273:143–149.

99    McGinnis JM, Foege WH. Actual causes of death in the United States. *JAMA* 1993;270:2207–2212.

100    Serenity Prayer. In: Brown RM, ed. *The Essential Reinhold Niebuhr; Selected Essays and Addresses*. New Haven, Conn.: Yale University Press, 1987.

## Chapter 9

1    Somers AR. Why not try preventing illness as a way of controlling Medicare costs? *N Engl J Med* 1985;311:853–856.

2    Satcher D. The prevention challenge and opportunity. *Health Affairs* 2006;25: 1009–1012.

3    Fineberg K. *Health Reform: Beyond Health Insurance*. President's Address, Institute of Medicine Annual Meeting, October 12, 2009.

4    Marshall E. Medicine under the microscope. *Science* 2009;326:1183–1185.

5    Bortz W. *Atherosclerosis*. Honors Thesis, Biology, Williams College, 1951.

6    Capewell S, Hayes D, Ford E, et al. Life years gained among U.S. adults from modern treatments and changes in the prevalence of six coronary heart disease risk factors between 1980 and 2000. *Am J Epidemiol* 2009;170:229–236.

7    Kottke T, Faith D, Jordan D, Pronk N, et al. Comparative effectiveness of heart disease prevention and treatment strategies. *Am J Prev Med* 2009;36:82–86.

8    Dzau VJ, Horiuchi M. Vascular remodeling: the emerging paradigm of programmed cell death (apoptosis). The Francis B. Parker Lectureship. *Chest* 1998;114:91S–99S.

9    Haskell W, Sims C, Myll J, Bortz W, et al. Coronary artery size and dilating capacity in ultradistance runners. *Circulation* 1993;87:1076–1082.

10    Horton R. Cancer: the malignant maneuver. *New York Review of Books*, March 2008.

11    Davis D. *The Secret History of the War on Cancer*. Philadelphia: Basic Books, 2007.

12    Willett W. Diet and cancer. *Oncologist* 2000;5:393–404.

13    Kogevinas M, Marmot M, Fox AJ, et al. Socioeconomic differences in cancer survival. *J Epidemiol Community Health* 1991;45:216–219.

14  Emerson H, Carson L. Diabetes mellitus, a contribution to its epidemiology based mainly on mortality statistics. *Ann Intern Med*, November 1924.

15  American Diabetes Association statistics, 2010.

16  Yale Diabetes Center Report, 2008.

17  American Diabetes Association Fact Sheet, 2010.

18  Bortz W. *Diabetes Danger*. New York: Select Books, 2005.

19  Couzin J. Bypassing medicine to treat diabetes. *Science* 2008;320:438–440.

20  Forbes.com. Obesity surgery complications on the decline. April 29, 2009.

21  Bortz W. The disuse syndrome. *West J Med* 1984;141:691–694.

22  Kraus H, Raab W. *Hypokinetic Disease: Disease Produced by the Lack of Exercise.* Springfield, Ill.: Charles C Thomas, 1991.

23  Booth FW. Sedentary death syndrome. *Am J Applied Physiol* 2004;29:447–462.

24  Knowler WC, Barrett-Connor E, Fowler SE, et al. Reduction in incidence of type II diabetes with lifestyle intervention or metformin. *N Engl J Med* 2002;348: 395–403.

25  Sledge CB. Structure, development and function of joints. *Orthop Clin North Am* 1975;6:619–628.

26  Bland JH. Reversibility of osteoarthritis: a review. *Am J Med* 1983;14:16–26.

27  Osteoporosis Foundation. *Clinician's Guide to Prevention and Treatment*, 2009.

28  Kivipelto M, Solomon A. Preventive neurology. *Neurology* 2009;73:168–169.

29  Fotuhi M, Hachinski V, Whitehouse P. Changing perspectives regarding late-life dementia. *Nature Reviews Neurology* 2009;5:649–658.

30  Baker L, Frank L, Foster-Schubert K, et al. Effects of aerobic exercise on mild cognitive impairment. *Neurology* 2010;67:71–79.

31  Nagahara AH, Merrill DA, Coppola G, et al. Neuroprotective effects of brain-derived neurotrophic factor in rodent and primate models of Alzheimer's disease. *Nature Medicine* 2009;15:331–337.

32  Cohen L, Chavez V, Chehimi J, eds. *Prevention Is Primary: Strategies for Community Well-Being*. San Francisco: Jossey Bass, 2007.

## Chapter 10

1  Cousins NC. Anatomy of an illness. *N Engl J Med* 1976;295:1458–1463.

2  Bortz WM, Barchas J, et al. Catecholamine, dopamine, and endorphin levels during extreme exercise. *N Engl J Med* 1981;315:466–467.

3  Juvenal Satires X. Wrong Desire is the Source of Suffering (100 ad).

4  Laslett P. *A Fresh Map of Life: The Emergence of the Third Age*. Cambridge, MA: Harvard University Press, 1991.

5  Schoenhofen EA, Wysznski DF, Andersen S, et al. Characteristics of 32 supercentenarians. *J Am Geriatr Soc* 2006;54:1237–1240.

6  Buettner D. *The Blue Zones: Lessons for Living Longer from the People Who Have Lived the Longest*. Washington DC: National Geographic Books, 2008.

7  The Island Where People Live Longer. *NPR Weekend Edition*, Saturday, May 2, 2009.

8   Leaf A. Search for the Oldest People. *National Geographic* 1973;143:93–119.

9   Farquhar J. *The American Way of Life Need Not be Dangerous to your Health.* Stanford: Stanford University Press, 1987.

10  Cumming E, Henry W. *Growing Old: The Process of Disengagement.* New York: Basic Books, 1961.

11  Carstensen LL, Fredrickson, BL. Influence of HIV status and age on cognitive representations of others. *Health Psychology* 1998;17:494–503.

12  Czikszentmihaly M. *Flow: The Psychology of Optimal Experience.* New York: Harper & Row, 1990.

13  Hu FB, Li TY, Colditz GA. Television watching and other sedentary behaviors in relation to risk of obesity and type II diabetes in women. *JAMA* 2003;289:1785–1791.

14  Perls T. The Different Pathways to Age 100. *Annals NY Acad Sci* 2005;1055:13–25.

15  Rowe J, Kahn R. Human aging: usual and successful. *Science* 1987;237:143–149.

16  Peterson P. *Gray Dawn: How the Age Wave Will Transform America and the World.* New York: Random House, 1999.

17  White KM. Longevity advances in high-income countries. *Population and Development Review* 2002;28:59–76.

18  Christensen K, Dublhammer G, Rau R, Vaupel JW. Ageing populations: the challenges ahead. *Lancet* 2009; Oct. 23:1196–1208.

19  Brody J. Healthy Aging, with Nary a Supplement. *New York Times*, Jan. 11, 2010.

20  Social Security Administration, Annual Report 2004.

21  Bortz W. Disuse and aging. *JAMA* 1982;248:1253–1258.

22  Bawden N. *Walking Naked.* New York: St. Martin's Press, 1981.

23  Cousins N. *Human Options.* New York: WW Norton, 1981.

24  Kashiwaya Y, Takeshima T, Mori N, Nakashima K, Clarke K, Veech RL. D-Beta-hydroxybutyrate protects neurons in models of Alzheimer's disease and Parkinson's disease. *Proc Natl Acad Sci USA* 2000;97:5440–5444.

25  McGinnis ML, Foege W. Actual causes of death. *JAMA* 1993;270:2207–2212.

26  Fried L, Tangen CM, Walston J, et al. The frailty phenotype. *J Geront A Biol Sci Med Sci* 2001;56:M146–156.

27  Bortz W. A conceptual framework of frailty; a review. *J Geron Med Sci* 2002; M283-M288.

28  Guralnik J, Ferrucci L, Simonsek G, et al. Lower extremity function over the age of 70 as a predictor of subsequent disability. *N Engl J Med* 1998;332:556–561.

29  Sheehan G. *Going the Distance: One Man's Journey to the End of his Life.* New York: Villard, 1996.

30  Hotchner AE. *Papa Hemingway.* New York: Carroll & Graf, 1999.

31  Kinsey A, Pomeroy W, Martin E. *Sexual Behavior in the Human Female.* Philadelphia: WB Saunders, 1953.

32  Masters W, Johnson V. *Human Sexual Response.* Boston: Little, Brown, 1970.

33  Comfort A. *The Joy of Sex.* New York: Simon & Schuster, 1972.

34  Lindau ST, Schumm LP, Lauman EO, et al. A study of sexuality and health among older adults in the United States. *N Engl J Med* 2007;357:762–774.

35  Jong E. *Fear of Fifty.* New York: Harper Collins, 1997.

36  Friedan B. *Fountain of Age*. New York: Touchstone, 1993.
37  Matheson B. *Ahead of the Curve: An Intimate Conversation with Women in the Second Half of Life*. Tucson: Wheatmark, 2009.
38  Yates LB, Djousse L, Kurth T, et al. Exceptional longevity in men: modifiable factors associated with survival and function to age 90. *Arch Intern Med* 2008;168: 284–290.
39  Smith GD, Frankel S, Yarnell J. Sex and death; are they related? Findings from the Caerphilly Cohort Study. *Br Med J* 1997;315:1641–1645.
40  Cleare AJ, Wessely SC. Just what the doctor ordered: more alcohol and sex [editorial]. *Br Med J* 1997;315:1641–1642.

## Chapter 11

1  Bortz WM. The trajectory of dying: functional state in the last year of life. *J Am Geriatrics Soc* 1990;30:146–150.
2  Fries JF. The compression of morbidity. *Millbank Mem Fund Q* 1983;61:397–419.
3  Socrates. Stanford Encyclopedia of Philosophy online. www.plato.stanford.edu
4  Epicurus. http://en.wikipedia.org/wiki/epicurus
5  Harris S. *The End of Faith: Religion, Terror, and the Future of Reason*. New York: WW Norton, 2004.
6  Cousins N. *Human Origins*. New York: WW Norton, 1981.
7  Santayana G. *Life of Reason*, quoted on www.Davebarry.com
8  Twain M. Quotes Uncertified. www.wikiquote.org.
9  Segerberg G. *Living to Be 100: 1200 Who Did It and How They Did It*. New York: Scribner, 1982.
10  Holmes OW. The Deacon's Masterpiece: or the Wonderful One Hoss Shay. From *The Autocrat of the Breakfast Table, 1857. The Complete Poetical Works of Oliver Wendell Holmes*. Boston: Houghton Mifflin, 1908.
11  Callahan D. *Setting Limits: Medical Goals in an Aging Society*. New York: Simon & Schuster, 1987.
12  Callahan D. *The Troubled Dream of Life: In Search of a Peaceful Death*. Touchstone, 1993.
13  Lamm R. *The Brave New World of Health Care*. Golden, Colo.: Fulcrum, 2003.
14  Tolstoi L. *The Death of Ivan Illyich and Master and Man*. New York: Random House, 1994.
15  Lynn J. Food and water can be withheld from dying patients; the very different situations of Claire Conroy and Karen Quinlan. *Death Educ* 1984;8:271–275.
16  Browning R. "Rabbi Ben Ezra." http://theotherpages.org/poems
17  Yalom I. *Staring at the Sun: Overcoming the Terror of Death*. San Francisco: Jossey Bass, 2008.
18  Thompson F. "The Mistress of Vision" (1913). http://www.poemhunter.com/quotations/famous.asp?people=Francis%20Thompson
19  Bortz W. *Dare to Be 100*. New York: Simon & Schuster, 1996.

## Chapter 12

1   Butler RN. Remarks, Annual Meeting of the American Geriatrics Society, 1987.
2   S. Brenner, Remarks, Stanford Symposium, 2004.
3   Kaiser Family Foundation December Health Tracking Poll, 12/2010.
4   Emanuel E, Fuchs V. *Healthcare Guaranteed: A Simple, Secure Solution for America.* New York: Public Affairs, 2009.
5   Orszag P. Demographics, access and costs: a federal perspective on health care policy and innovation. Stanford Conference: Better Health, Lower Cost: Can Innovation Save Health Reform? September 16, 2008.
6   Arrow K. Uncertainty and the welfare economics of medical care. *American Economics Review*, 1963.
7   Savedoff WD. Kenneth Arrow and the birth of health economics. *Bulletin WHO* 2004;42:139–140.
8   Christensen C, Grossman JH, Hwang J. *The Innovators' Prescription: A Disruptive Solution for Health Care.* New York: McGraw Hill, 2009.
9   Grove A. Left Shift, Address at Stanford University, Nov. 2, 2006.
10  Orszag P. *New Ideas About Human Behavior in Economics and Medicine.* Marshall Seidman Lecture, Harvard Medical School, October 2008.
11  Sen A. Capitalism beyond the crisis. *New York Review of Books*, March 26, 2009.
12  Reich R. *Supercapitalism; The Transformation of Business, Democracy, and Everyday Life.* New York: Random House, 2007.
13  Sox H. *Annals of Internal Medicine*'s Harold Sox, MD, discusses Physicians Charter of Professionalism. Interview by B Vastag. *JAMA* 2001;286:3065–3066.
14  Brody H. Medicine's ethical responsibility for health care reform: the top five list. *N Engl J Med* 2010;362:283–285.
15  Bishop G, Brodkey AC. Personal responsibility and physician responsibility: West Virginia's Medicaid plan. *N Engl J Med* 2006;355:756–758.
15A Wall Street Journal "Many Americans Back Higher Costs for People with Unhealthy Lifestyles" July 19, 2002.
16  Fahrenthold DA. Mass. bill requires health coverage. *Washington Post*, April 5, 2006.
17  Enthoven AC. *Curing Fragmentation with Integrated Delivery Systems.* Charles Sills Lecture, Harvard Law School, June 8, 2008.
18  Aristotle. *Nichomachean Ethics.* Oxford World Classics, 1980.
19  Dostoevsky F. *The Brothers Karamazov* (1880). New York: Bantam, 1970.
20  Plato. *Republic* (380 BC). Indianapolis: Hackett, 1992.
21  Bell D. *The Cultural Contradictions of Capitalism.* New York: Basic Books, 1976.
22  Aquinas T. *History of Political Economy,* Vol. 32, Fall 2000.
23  Halvorson G. Health care delivery innovation perspective. Stanford Conference: Better Health, Lower Cost: Can Innovation Save Health Reform? September 16, 2008.
24  Rawls J. *A Theory of Justice.* Cambridge, Mass.: Harvard University Press, 1971.
25  Berlin I. *Liberty.* Oxford, UK: Oxford University Press, 2000.
26  Hardin G. Tragedy of the commons. *Science* 1968;162:1243–1248.

27  Madison J. *The Federalist no. 51*: The structure of the government must furnish the proper checks and balance between the different departments. Feb. 6, 1788.

28  Hegel GF. A historian looks at Hegel. www.Historicalinsights.com/dave/hegel

29  Lincoln A. Essay 1854, quoted in http://www.blueoregon.com/2009/02/lincoln-on-government/

30  Hiatt HH. Protecting the medical commons; who is responsible? *N Engl J Med* 1975;293:228–235.

31  Cassel CK, Brennan TE. Managing medical resources: return to the commons? *JAMA* 2007;297:2518–2521.

32  Siegler M. The progression from physician paternalism to patient autonomy to bureaucratic parsimony. *Arch Intern Med* 1985;145:713–715.

33  Stewart A, Ware J. *Measuring and Monitoring Quality of Life in Populations*. Durham, NC: Duke University Press, 1992.

34  Debley T, Stewart J. *The Story of Sidney Garfield: The Visionary Who Turned Sick Care into Health Care*. Portland, Oregon: Permanente Press, 2009.

35  Dobzhansky T. Nothing in biology makes any sense except in the light of evolution. *American Biology Teacher* 1973;35:125–129.

36  Will G. Corn-fed nation. *Washington Post*, March 6, 09.

37  Pollan M. *In Defense of Food: An Eater's Manifesto*. New York: Penguin Books, 2008.

38  www.forbes.com, September 15, 2005

39  Pronk N, Goodman MJ, O'Connor PJ. Relation between modifiable health risks and short-term health care charges. *JAMA* 1999;282:2235–2238.

40  Edington D. Opportunities to improve care and manage costs for employees with chronic diseases. *Managed Care Interface,* Supplement C, 2003:5–7.

41  Breslow L. Survey methods in general populations: studies in a total community. Alameda and Contra Costa Counties, California. *Milbank Mem Fund Q* 1965;43: 317–325.

42  Blair SN, Kohl HW, Paffenbarger RS, et al. Physical fitness and all-cause mortality; a prospective study of healthy men and women. *JAMA* 1989;262:2305–2401.

## Chapter 13

1  Robert Wood Johnson Foundation Annual Report, 2009.

2  Stewart A, Verboncoeur CJ, McClellan BT, et al. Physical activity outcomes of CHAMP II; a physical activity promotion program for older adults. *J Geron A Biol Sci Med Sci* 2001;56:M465–M470.

3  Gardner J. "John Gardner: UnCommon American." Film, PBS Classroom.

4  Bortz W. Memo to John Gardner, Community Health Planning, January 12, 2001.

5  Puska P, Stahl T. Health in all policies: the Finnish initiative; background, principles and current issues. *Ann Rev Public Health* 2010 [e-pub Jan 4].

6  Lavizzo-Mourey R, McGinnis JM. Making the case for active living communities. *Am J Pub Health* 2003;93:1386–1388.

7   Sondik ET, Huang DT, Klein RJ, Satcher D. Progress toward the 2010 goals and objectives. *Ann Rev Pub Health* [e-pub Dec. 1, 2009].

8   Robertson A. Reflections on the politics of need. In Callahan D. *Promoting Healthy Behavior: How Much Freedom? Whose Responsibility?* Washington, DC: Georgetown University Press, 2007.

9   Ratey J. *Spark.* New York: Little Brown, 2008.

10  Marcus MB. Town sets off on healthy path practicing 4 keys to longevity. *USA Today* June 15, 2009.

11   Report: Crimes of the heart. *Newsweek* February 15, 2010.

12  Eiberg S, Hasselstrom H, Gronveldt V, et al. Maximum oxygen uptake and objectively measured physical activity in Danish children 6–7 years of age: The Copenhagen School Child Intervention Study 2004. *Br J Sports Med* 2005;39:725–730.

13  www.Saludthefilm.net, 2006.

14  Wood PD, Haskell W, Klein H, et al. Distribution of plasma lipoproteins in middle-aged runners. *Metabolism* 1976;25:1249–1256.

15  Chakravarty EF, Hubert HB, Lingala VB, Fries JF. Reduced disability and mortality among aging runners: a 21-year longitudinal study. *Arch Intern Med* 2008;168: 1638–1646.

16  Chenowith D, Hollander M, Bortz W. The cost of sloth: using a tool to measure the cost of physical inactivity. *Health and Fitness Journal* 2006;10:1–8.

17  Bandura A. *Self-Efficacy: The Exercise of Control.* New York: Worth, 1997.

18  Farquhar J, Fortmann SP, Flora JA, et al. Effects of community-wide education on cardiovascular risk factors; the Stanford 5 City Project. *JAMA* 1990;264:359–365.

19  Rogacheva A, Laatikainen T, Tossavainen K, et al. Changes in cardiovascular risk factors among adolescents from 1995–2004 in the Republic of Karelia, Russia. *Eur J Public Health* 2007;17:257–262.

20  Enthoven AC, van de Ven WP. Going Dutch: managed competition health insurance in the Netherlands. *N Engl J Med* 2007;357:2421–2425.

21  Olshansky SJ, Goldman DP, Zheng Y, et al. Aging in America in the 21st century: demographic forecasts from the MacArthur Foundation Research Network on an Aging Society. *Milbank Mem Fund Q* 2009;87:842–862.

22  Kilmer G, Roberts H, Li Y, et al. MMWR Surveillance summary, 2008.

23  News release: Well-being in the U.S. continues its downward trend in December: five of six sub-measures drop year over year. Gallup Healthways Report, January 14, 2010.

24  CDC State Obesity Rates, 2009.

25  Knowler WC, Barrett-Conner E, Fowler SE, et al. Reduction in the incidence of type II diabetes with lifestyle intervention or metformin. *N Engl J Med* 2002;346: 393–403.

26  Dustman RE, Ruhling RO, Russell EM, et al. Aerobic exercise training and improved neuropsychological function of older individuals. *Neurobiol Aging* 1984;5:35–45.

27  Sallis RE. Exercise is medicine and physicians need to prescribe it. *Br J Sports Med* 2009;43:3–4.

## Afterword

1 Dubos R. Hippocrates in modern dress. In: Sobel D, ed. *Ways of Health*. New York: Harcourt Brace Jovanovich, 1979.

2 Gardner J. *National Renewal*. http://www.independentsector.org/about_john_gardner.

# Index

238    Index